P9-DSZ-108

MVFOL

Believe It,
Be It

Believe It, Be It

How Being
THE BIGGEST LOSER
WON ME BACK MY LIFE

Ali Vincent

This book is intended as a reference volume only, not as a medical manual. The information given here is designed to help you make informed decisions about your health. It is not intended as a substitute for any treatment that may have been prescribed by your doctor. If you suspect that you have a medical problem, we urge you to seek competent medical help.

Mention of specific companies, organizations, or authorities in this book does not imply endorsement by the author or publisher, nor does mention of specific companies, organizations, or authorities imply that they endorse this book, its author, or the publisher.

Internet addresses and telephone numbers given in this book were accurate at the time it went to press.

Rodale books may be purchased for business or promotional use or for special sales. For information, please write to: Special Markets Department, Rodale Inc., 733 Third Avenue, New York, NY 10017

Printed in the United States of America
Rodale Inc. makes every effort to use acid-free ♾, recycled paper ♻.

Book design by Robin Black
Photographs on pages 1, 13, and 23 are courtesy of the author. All others are by NBC Universal Photo.

Library of Congress Cataloging-in-Publication Data

Vincent, Ali.
    Believe it, be it : how being the biggest loser won me back my life / Ali Vincent.
        p.   cm.
    Includes bibliographical references.
    ISBN-13 978–1–60529–548–0   hardcover
    ISBN-13 978–1–60529–412–4   paperback
    1. Vincent, Ali—Health.   2. Weight loss—United States—Biography.   3. Overweight women—United States—Biography.   4. Biggest loser (Television program).   I. Title.
    RM222.2V527   2009
    613.2'5092—dc22
    [B]   2009036835

Distributed to the trade by Macmillan
2   4   6   8   10   9   7   5   3   1   paperback

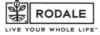

We inspire and enable people to improve their lives and the world around them.

To my mom, Bette-Sue Burklund. I love you with all that I am and all that I hope to become. Thank you for loving me and giving so much of who you are to create and mold the person I am today. Without you there would be no me. Forever I will draw on the moments of laughter and joy that you, Amber, and I shared in the many drive-thrus singing, "Don't you turn my brown eyes blue." You have always been my light.

Contents

Acknowledgments

I would like to thank and express my love to my family for always believing in me. Thanks to my mom, Bette-Sue, for being willing to put herself out there so that I could have the courage to do the same, and her husband, Richard, for balancing my mom. To my dad, John, for exemplifying that you can create what you want, and my stepmom, Peggy, for showing me that you only get better with age. To my grandparents, Florence and Cordon, for loving Amber and me and making sure we always had someone there. My aunt Judi who loved us as her own and whom I miss daily. My sister Amber, who has always been my constant and who has shown me that you can give your heart to someone else without losing yourself, and her husband, Brian, whom I love dearly. My younger sister, Holly, and her husband, Andy, for their continued and unconditional love and support. My brothers, Joey and Adam, for keeping it real and kicking my butt every chance they get. My nieces Alexandra, Alexis, Avery, Macy, and Madison and my nephew, McCoy, for inspiring me to live and love to the best of my ability.

To *all* my friends (you know who you are), I love you and thank you for always being there for me.

To Jillian Michaels and Bob Harper, thank you for helping me see the light that has always been inside me and showing me how to fan it into a roaring fire again. I love you both madly.

Thank you to Mark Koops, Chad Bennett, Ben Silverman, Dave Broome, JD Roth, Todd A. Nelson, and all the cast and crew of Season 5's *The Biggest Loser*. I am truly grateful to each and every one of you for providing me the opportunity and encouragement to create my destiny. And special thanks to the two castmates who have become a part of my life: Brittany Aberle and Mark Kruger.

I also want to thank Alison Sweeney for being able to connect with me and push me personally to do more than even I knew I was capable of. You continue to inspire me to create. I look forward to a lifetime of friendship and making a difference together, one person at a time.

To Sidney Griffin, Melissa DeLuca, Tony Wells, Carl Liebert, and the whole team from 24 Hour Fitness, I love being part of the 24 Hour family. Thank you for helping me fulfill my dream of touching the lives of people just like me. And to Janine Drake, David Jenkins, Tom Oliver, Tex Prows, and the team from Designer Whey Protein for helping me educate and get the message out there.

A special thanks to my editor at Rodale, Julie Will, who suggested I write this book after a simple conversation. Thank you for initiating this and putting in countless hours to make *Believe It, Be It* happen. And thank you to Andy Barzvi at ICM, who guided me through this process. She's been excited to help me share my story from day 1. Well, we finally did it!

I would like to thank Melissa Roberson whom I fell in love with from the first day that Mom and I met her while trying on our Biggest Loser sports bras and biker shorts! I cannot think of another person in this world with whom I'd rather partake in this journey. Your laughter and pure compassion has allowed me the space to dig deep, knowing that I was safe to just be me.

And last, but certainly not least, thanks to all of the fans who support and who encourage me daily to continue on this journey. Together we can change the world by loving and taking care of ourselves first. Remember: Believe It, Be It . . . I do.

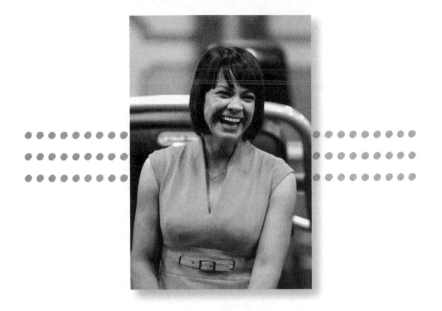

Introduction

My name is Ali Vincent, and I am the Biggest Loser. I still love saying it. Sometimes I'm in the shower and I think to myself, "I'm the first female Biggest Loser!" It's something I will feel wonderful about for the rest of my life, and it's an accomplishment that fuels all of my future goals.

In October 2007, when I officially joined the Season 5 cast of NBC's hit show *The Biggest Loser*, I weighed 234 pounds. About 6 months later, on April 15, 2008, I weighed 122 pounds. In a finale broadcast live to millions of people, I stepped onto a giant scale and registered a total weight loss of 112 pounds—and became the first woman ever to win the show's grand prize. I had lost 47.86 percent of my starting weight—nearly half of me had vanished.

But honestly, before I stepped on that scale, I felt that I had already won. By shedding those pounds and by confronting the emotional issues that had led to my weight gain, I had also won a whole new life. One that felt open and full of hope, almost newly born. And I think everyone can have that feeling. I know everyone *deserves* to have that feeling.

Since winning the show, I've traveled across the country, meeting with and talking to people who want to reclaim their lives. They are struggling to lose their excess weight and all the other burdens and hurts they've been carrying around that keep them from realizing their dreams. My story is about weight loss, sure, but it's also about coming back to life, emerging from a place of darkness and isolation. And I know there are others who share the very same struggles, who want so much more for themselves, and who have so much more to give to others than they can currently offer. They are the reasons why I wrote this book. I've learned a lot on this journey that I want to share with others and that I hope will help others. I truly believe we can change the world one person at a time.

This is the story of how I changed my life, a story of personal struggle and triumph. It's the story of how I began to dream big, get healthy, and allow myself to start thinking, "Why *not* me?"

ABOUT MY BELL

A friend once gave me the gift of a little bell with a ribbon attached to the top that said, "Dream It, Be It." I packed the bell in my suitcase when my mom and I traveled to California for the final casting selection for *The Biggest Loser*. One day, when we were sitting in our hotel room, I took it out and started shaking it and having a little fun with my mom, saying, "Believe it, be it." At the time, I was joking around—I had never really understood the idea of having a mantra or creating an intention for your life. But the more I kept ringing that bell and saying, "Believe it, be it," the more it felt right. And from that moment on, I began to think and feel that I could do it. That not only would I be selected for the show, but I could win it and become the first female Biggest Loser.

When we were selected for the show, I took the bell with me to *The Biggest Loser* ranch. I used to ring it and repeat my mantra every night before bed and every morning when I woke up. At the end of our season, when I was a finalist, the producers wanted to create a time capsule for the next season and plant it somewhere on campus. They asked all of us to donate something that could be included in it. My immediate thought was that I would give them my bell. But I got nervous. "Oh my God," I thought, "I can't give up my bell. That's my *bell*." But when I really thought about it, I realized I didn't need it anymore. Because I believed it, and I had become what I wanted to be. I am it. I thought of the bell as a torch I needed to pass.

So I put my bell in the time capsule with a handwritten note advising its recipient to stay present, to stay conscious, and to always know where they were going so that they could get there and achieve their goals. And I shared the story of my bell, saying that it helped me become the first female Biggest Loser. Of course, at the time, I hadn't won anything. But I believed it would happen, and I wrote in my note that this little bell had helped me become the person I knew I could be.

In the end, the producers didn't use the bell for the time capsule. Many months later, I returned to campus to guest host an episode of the show when host Alison Sweeney was having her baby. I asked one of the crew members if they still had my bell. They found it and returned it to me, and today it hangs in my kitchen. I still look at it every day and say, "Believe it, be it." I've always thought that if anyone ever needed my bell, if it would help give them strength, I'd give it to them. I'd pass it along. In a way, my story is that bell. My hope is that in sharing my story, I can help you believe in yourself, and help you become whatever it is that you want to be.

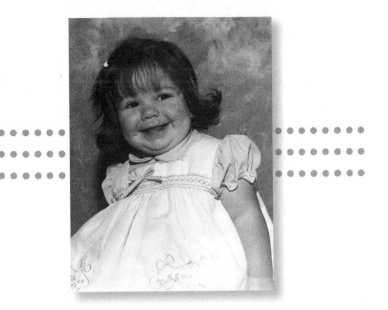

ONE

Where Change Begins

*The only battle to win is the battle within,
that place where we realize that we deserve to
have and create all that we want in our lives.*

Somewhere between childhood and adulthood, I lost my way. I lost my dreams, my hopes, my goals, my happiness, my sense of self. It even felt as though I lost my family and my friends. I didn't want to go out, didn't want to see any of the people I loved—because I was afraid they would be able to see how bad I felt about myself. I didn't like

• 1

myself, and I didn't have the courage to admit that to myself, much less admit it to my friends. I was living a life of complacency. Checked out. Shut down.

One thing I *wasn't* losing was weight. In fact, by the time I hit my early thirties, I was up to about 234 pounds on a 5-foot-5 frame. At one point in my life, I had been a world-class athlete, a nationally ranked synchronized swimmer. I had been athletic and popular in high school, a "trophy" girlfriend, a cheerleader. I'd had dreams of doing something big, of making a difference, especially in the lives of women. From the age of 6 or 7, I distinctly remember telling my mom that I was going to help women when I grew up. I always felt that women didn't get the same breaks that men did, that life was handed to them differently. But now I couldn't even help myself.

This is the story of my journey back to myself. Back to the Ali who had dreams of making a difference in the lives of others and living life on a larger scale. And what a journey it has turned out to be. It's taken me to places I never imagined I would go, including a reality weight-loss TV show called *The Biggest Loser,* where I struggled, sweated, and cried in front of millions of viewers while wearing a sports bra and bike shorts. Oh, and I did this with my mom, the unforgettable Bette-Sue, who the entire nation learned was never shy about expressing an opinion. Mom would end up being my partner in weight loss, and we would cover some painful emotional history between us—all on camera, no less.

I grew up in a family of beautiful women, all of whom made

a huge impression on me and all of whom struggled with their weight. As a kid, I wouldn't even have known my mom was heavy, except that she said she was fat. She tried everything she could think of to lose weight—she took diet pills and went on every weird diet in the world, all with the blessing of my grandmother, Florence Alison (after whom I'm named). Grandma grew up in New Zealand and came to the United States at the age of 20. My mom's sister, my aunt Judi, died of obesity-related cancer. Weight was a major topic of discussion when I was growing up, for all of us except my sister, Amber. She never had a weight problem—a huge source of frustration for me when I started to pile on the pounds in my late teens.

Even though my story was watched by millions of viewers as a weight loss journey—gaining it, losing it, trying to keep it off— my journey is a lot bigger than what you saw on TV. Because behind weight gain are the larger hurts and questions that have to be explored, probed, and understood before weight loss and maintenance is a possibility. It's a bigger issue than just calories in, calories out. There's something fundamental you have to understand about yourself before you can change your life for good. The trick is, it's different for every person. You have to figure out your stuff, just like I did mine. But maybe by sharing my story, I can help you understand yours. I certainly know the pain, deprivation, and insecurity that come with a life of obesity. But I also know there's a much richer, fuller life waiting for all of us. And that if you can believe in yourself, you can become your best possible self.

"WHY ARE YOU FAT?"

Working out with my trainer, Jillian Michaels, on *The Biggest Loser* ranch one day, I was struggling and sweating with the pullup machine, feeling as vulnerable as can be, when she suddenly asked me, "Why are you here?"

"Because I'm fat," I answered.

Jillian took it a step further and responded, "Why are you fat?"

I knew what she was getting at. I'd been just kind of letting life happen to me—I didn't feel worthy of wanting anything more for myself. And I'd had those feelings for a long time. When we started out at the ranch, Jillian asked everyone to write down a list of reasons why we were there. My first one was "I have always felt alone." My fat protected me and gave me a reason for people leaving me. Because, otherwise, why would they go? What was so bad about me? The fat gave me a reason—it justified my feelings of loneliness.

• •

NO MORE EXCUSES

When we really take a moment to look at it, who are we really excusing when we make excuses? And how do they help us? They don't. It took me a while to understand this, and quite frankly I am still grasping the idea. This is how I think of it: I have to be proud of the choices I make and forgive myself for the not-so-good ones. Making excuses is not going to get me any closer to my goals.

• •

GROWING UP MORMON

I weighed more than 9 pounds when I was born. My mom had big babies. By the time I was 4 months old, I was so fat I looked plastic. I looked as if I was going to pop.

I had a pretty dramatic childhood. I don't blame anybody—when I look back on it, I think everyone was doing the best they could to raise me and my older sister, Amber. She and I never wanted for anything, other than a stable, ordered family life. And, unfortunately, the fact that we didn't have one was made even more obvious by the fact that everyone else around us did.

I grew up in Mesa, Arizona, in a community with a strict moral code based on the Church of Jesus Christ of Latter-Day Saints—Mormonism. I can't emphasize enough how important a role the church played in how I felt I was supposed to be and act and what kind of family I thought I was supposed to have. I grew up thinking that you were supposed to have both a mom and dad

• •

LEARN TO SAY NO

Sometimes it seems like women are good at giving to everyone but themselves. If you're going to get healthy, you're going to have to take care of yourself. And that means saying no to some requests for your time and attention—time and attention you may need to devote to planning, grocery shopping, cooking, working out, or resting.

• •

who raised their kids at home, your mom and dad weren't supposed to drink or smoke, no one was supposed to have sex before marriage, and you weren't supposed to associate with anyone who did those things. That's what I learned in Sunday school.

But here's what I had: divorced parents: a dad who was Catholic, Mexican, and rarely around; and a mom who smoked, drank, partied, had lots of boyfriends, and wasn't exactly your typical stay-at-home mom. It was all very confusing for a little Mormon girl.

My parents had divorced by the time I was 2. I have no memories of my dad living with us. Mom was a cheerleader in high school and hung out with a non-Mormon crowd. My dad, John Vincent, wasn't exactly what a couple of Mormon parents would have chosen for their daughter, but after she got pregnant with Amber, they married.

My grandparents did the daily work of raising us. My mom, Amber, and I lived with them most of the time. Sometimes my mom would find an apartment and we'd move out for a little while, but we always ended up back with Grandma and Grandpa. Our grandparents got us to school, drove us to all of our activities. They made sure we had everything we needed. But I still knew I wasn't like everyone else. I knew I didn't fit in. I felt like I wore a scarlet letter that separated me from all the other kids.

I remember going on a school camping trip in fifth grade. I was so excited because my mom had volunteered to be a chaperone, something her work schedule rarely allowed her to do. Some of the kids wanted to play a prank on her by putting a dead fish in her purse. But when they opened it, they found a pack of cigarettes. That was a pretty serious offense to a bunch of Mormon kids, and I was so embarrassed. They taunted me and told me that I was going to be drinking and smoking by the time I was in junior high. I felt so shamed by that kind of talk. But as I got older, it would fuel my own rebellions. I would give them something to talk about, all right.

My grandparents were active members of the Mormon church and didn't approve of Mom's lifestyle, but they couldn't do much to stop her. I always felt conflicted about my mom. I loved that she was pretty, that she was the life of the party, but I didn't love being pulled out of my bunk bed at night when she came home drunk and got into a fight with my grandparents. Amber and I were the pawns in that relationship. If Mom got mad enough, she'd threaten to take us away from them. I also didn't love being

• •

DON'T SHOULDER OTHERS' OPINIONS

Don't surround yourself with people whose opinions make you feel bad about yourself. As I began to lose weight and feel better, I realized that if I was going to keep certain people in my life, I needed to talk to them. If I didn't appreciate the way they made jokes about me or commented on my actions, I let them know. I stand up for myself now, more than I ever have in my life.

• •

thrust into the middle of the fights she would have with boy-friends, because she knew a grown man wouldn't hit a little girl. I was supposed to protect her.

Some of those boyfriends weren't exactly the best picks. One had been in prison. One stole from us. Another guy, a big biker guy, used to visit in the middle of the night. Sometimes I would run into him in the hallway, and I was terrified—he was enormous. It never occurred to me—or Mom—that he was married until we saw him years later with his wife. I think that's just how discon-nected Mom was from her actions at that time. She was struggling with her own demons and worthiness when it came to dating.

But even amid all this chaos, I still knew my mom loved me. When Mom got us ready for school, she always gave our ponytails curls and ribbons and dressed us in matching outfits. She would cut our hair and perm it and braid it so tightly and perfectly, it would change the way our faces looked. One Christmas she worked an extra job as a waitress just to buy bikes for my sister and me. I don't think she was such a good waitress—she spilled things, didn't get orders right—but all the customers loved her. Everyone always loved my mom, though she didn't love herself.

I think everyone in our family tried hard to make up for the fact that we were two little girls with no dad at home. If any-thing, we were given too much. Amber and I caught on at an early age: If one adult wouldn't give us what we wanted, we'd just move to the next. We weren't taught to save money. We didn't have chores. I don't remember having to clean my room or make my bed. We learned very little about personal responsibility.

When my dad remarried and had his own family, my mom hated the idea of sharing Amber and me with them. It made it hard for me to form relationships with my stepfamily. I was also sad that all of my half-siblings had a mom *and* my dad. Why did they get to have a family and I didn't?

But my mom brought out the protector in me. I wanted to defend her. She could be loud and outspoken, and she could make me cringe, but I also knew she was gossiped about in our community, that her actions attracted the judgment of others—and I hated that. When she went to church with us on occasion, she would pass up the sacrament because even though she lived life her way, she was Mormon enough not to take the sacrament when her body was not a temple.

As I hit my teen years, I started acting out. I drank, I hung out with a faster crowd, and I lost my virginity in a public park when I was 13. I felt like people thought I was a bad kid anyway, so I might as well become one. I was definitely not living the Mormon life. In fact, I was turning into my mother, and though I loved her, I didn't want her life. I was becoming a woman who didn't value her body.

MOVE ON AND DREAM BIG

When you feel so lost, it's hard to see that there is potential to have a better life one day, let alone understand that everything you need to create that life is already right inside of you.

• •

IT'S ABOUT YOU

Sometimes on the ranch, it seemed like success was about proving something to someone else, winning at any cost. But I don't know if that lays the foundation for permanent change in your life. For me, it was important to understand that I was losing weight for me, to get healthy to create a better life. When I realized that, it was liberating. The power to succeed or fail was up to me and only me.

• •

In order to have any chance of success, I've learned that you have to accept yourself and let go of the past failures or weaknesses that have been holding you back. It's important to look forward, not backward—to get really clear on your future and what *you* want it to be. It's not written in stone. Once you know what you want your life to look like, you can figure out how to make it happen.

Every season on *The Biggest Loser,* we see contestants open themselves up, heart and soul, for the world to see and judge—all because they want a chance to change their lives. Many of them, like me, lost touch with themselves somewhere along the way as they gained the weight. Others have been spending so much time and energy taking care of others that they haven't been taking care of themselves. And then there are those who have been overweight all their lives and simply don't know how to get healthy. Everyone has a story.

Each season, *The Biggest Loser* allows a few lucky contestants to take a break from their day-to-day lives so that they can focus on themselves and learn how to end their self-destructive habits. But you don't have to be on the show to experience a change—I think all of us who watch the show and allow these people into our living rooms can relate to their struggles, and we all exult in their successes. *The Biggest Loser* ranch is a place where people reinvent themselves. As contestants, some of us start to remember who we used to be, and some of us get the opportunity for the first time in our lives to show the world who we have always known we could be. In either case, we are never the same afterward.

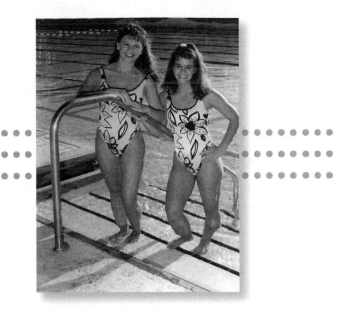

TWO

Living a Small Life

*There was a part of me always beating myself up.
I knew I was supposed to be living a bigger life
than I was. I was living a small life. It wasn't a
bad life by any means, but I was supposed to
make a bigger difference, and I knew that from
the time I was a little girl.*

I swam before I walked. Grandma was a swimmer in New
Zealand, and Mom was a nationally ranked speed swimmer. When I was little, we'd play "little duckies" in the
pool. My mom, Amber, and I would swim like ducks in a

row, and I was always the last little ducky behind Amber, farthest from my mom, which I hated! But I loved the water from the start. I knew I belonged there (I'm a Pisces), and I created my own world, pretending I was a mermaid.

I started out speed swimming in summer leagues, and the coaches of those teams created a synchronized swimming team. Amber and I were invited to join the Arizona Aqua Stars, and I became a member of a year-round team by the age of 6. The pool was my world. I had my safe place down there under the water, a place I got to create and live in. I was convinced that I was a mermaid, so much so that I believed I didn't need to come up for air. I'd just let my face barely break the surface of the water and take in a little gulp of air as I dolphin-dived my way back under. My coach would peer into the depths of the pool, shouting, "Ali, where are you?" The thing I loved most about my mermaid life was that I got to decide when I would surface.

We had swim practice every morning and afternoon. Grandma woke us up and took us to 5:00 a.m. practice. When we grew older, we'd ride our bikes to practice, and she'd follow behind us in the car. After school, I never played with friends—I went to the pool.

Synchronized swimming was for me the best of all worlds— I gained the endurance of a swimmer, the flexibility of a gymnast, the poise of a dancer, *and* I got to be in the water. Little did I know that, years later, I'd be too ashamed to get in a swimsuit.

WHEN THE POUNDS APPEARED

In high school, I stopped synchronized swimming and became more socially involved in school and activities. I was on the fast track to high school popularity as Amber's little sister. I even became a cheerleader. Yet I still felt a little different from the rest of the crowd. People knew me, yet they didn't. It didn't help that during my three years of high school (I graduated with a GED), I attended five different schools as Amber and I moved back and forth between our parents' houses. I identified with the outcasts, the people who didn't fit in. If I saw someone eating lunch by themselves, I'd go sit with them, and my friends knew better than to question me about it. I still liked being a cute cheerleader and a trophy girlfriend, but no one messed with me.

When I was swimming, I could eat whatever I wanted, and I didn't even think about it. I could eat an entire pizza. But I had grown so used to fueling my body as an athlete that when I quit swimming, my appetite stayed the same. And at that point in my life, I hadn't made the connection that what I was eating could change my body. I didn't think of food in terms of calories or fuel.

I didn't really understand exercise, either. I had taken dance classes and had done weight training, but that was part of the swimming program. And I didn't think of swimming as exercise. It was a passion, something I enjoyed. But my body knew it was exercise, and when I stopped, some pounds started to creep on.

I gained those first 5 pounds around the time I was 18, just out of high school. And the weird thing is, I thought of myself as obese. My trophy girlfriend status started to slip, and I remember feeling like one boyfriend didn't love me anymore not because of who I was, but because of the weight I was gaining. I wanted to be loved for myself, not just how I looked. But it didn't feel like things were turning out that way.

No one said anything to me, but I was starting to feel uncomfortable in my own skin. I have a very clear memory of being pulled over by a police officer after I first started gaining weight, and when I gave him my license—which listed my weight—he said, "No way you're 150 pounds." And I remember thinking, "You're right; I'm probably more." Because of my athletic build, people underestimated my weight. When I heard friends complaining about what they weighed, I would think, "If only they knew." My sister, Amber, managed to stay fit after we quit swimming, which made my weight gain even harder.

• •

GET READY FOR FEELINGS

For years I unconsciously tried to fill voids in my life with food. Once I was no longer doing that, I had to deal with the emotions that were causing me to overeat in the first place. But as my mom once said, it gets a lot easier to deal with life's curveballs when you're not hiding under layers of fat. It's not easy breaking down the walls that have protected us from life—but those walls have also stopped us from living the lives we truly want.

• •

• •

NO FAST AND EASY

Before *The Biggest Loser,* I was a fast-food junkie. On the ranch, I learned there are several steps to making a healthy meal. There's weighing the food, preparing the food. . . . I wanted fast and easy, but then I remembered that fast and easy is what got me to 234 pounds.

• •

In my mind, I was huge. After the first 5 pounds, I *felt* huge. Then I felt huge at 150 . . . 160 . . . 170. As the numbers got bigger, I just got disconnected from them. I started to withdraw. In fact, I avoided having my picture taken so much that when I got to *The Biggest Loser* and they asked me for pictures from the past few years, I didn't have any to give them. I was a fat girl, and fat girls don't have their picture taken. I hadn't documented my life because I didn't want to look at it.

I started trying diet pills and various weight loss programs. I'd always lose 10 pounds in 2 weeks, then I'd gradually stop going to meetings or paying attention to the rules. It was too much discipline for me. I didn't make it a point to understand how my body worked. I just did what they told me to do for a while, and then I'd gradually lose interest and gain the weight right back.

LEARNING ON THE JOB

Eventually I found myself at a community college in a small town I didn't like. It was very Mormon, and I wasn't feeling too Mormon.

Good Mormon girls don't have sex, and, well, I wasn't a good Mormon girl in that regard. I wasn't going to school very often, either.

I worked odd jobs. I was a waitress in a lot of fast-food places and chain restaurants, and I ate at work. I felt bad about myself and gradually stopped going out socially. But I did work hard. My first job was at a pizza parlor, and I had burns up and down my arms because I made sure there was not one single bubble in those pizzas. Whether it was making pizzas or sweeping floors, my work was important to me. Somehow at my job, I could show excellence and control. It was a way for me to be acknowledged in my life because I wasn't showing up anywhere else.

During one of my fading relationships, I moved to Texas and worked in a glass factory. It was hot, dirty, intense work, handling huge plates of glass. The first day I showed up in full makeup, which melted off my face within minutes. I worked alongside grown men, some of whom would quit after their first shift, the work was so grueling. How had I ended up a factory girl? I'd never been in a factory in my life. But I kept myself going by thinking about the next break during my shift. If I could just last until that break, and the next, then I could make it through the day. (It's a strategy I would use later, when I was struggling on the treadmill at *The Biggest Loser* ranch.) And I would think about my grandparents. They were my safety net if my life started falling apart. If things got really horrible, I knew I could call Grandpa. But standing next to the heat of that glass furnace, I also started to think about what I really wanted in my life.

I realized that I wanted to be a hairstylist.

I had always loved it; I'd wanted to do hair from the time I was a little girl. I used to get out of swim practice early so I could use a butane-operated curling iron, called at that time a "clicker," on my coach's hair. I braided all of my teammates' hair for award ceremonies when Amber and I were synchronized swimmers. I think I learned from my mom, who always cut our hair, gave us perms, and did everything else she could to style our hair in the latest trends. She was just naturally good at it, and it turned out I was, too.

But there I was in a glass factory in Texas. I became a small-parts cutter, and one day I got injured. That was it for me. I packed up my car and went home.

I knew going to beauty school would be hard. I had bills to pay. So I applied for and received financial aid, worked three jobs, and went to school. I was determined to go to the best school I could find. I went to school all day. Then at night I worked as a waitress. On my weekends, I got up at 4:30 a.m. to work the breakfast/lunch shift in a restaurant, and then evenings I worked as a cocktail waitress at a bar. At beauty school, I waxed the floors to earn an extra $50.

BECOMING A STYLIST

I loved becoming a stylist. I loved how I could make a client look, of course, but also I loved the relationship, how much the client trusted me. That person sitting in your chair is giving you permission to create the image they present to the world. I felt good about helping people feel good about themselves. Once someone became my client, they would return.

And I was pretty confident in my skills—I thought of myself as an artist. I was heavy, and I didn't dress the part in terms of wearing form-fitting, trendy clothes, but my looser, plus-size wardrobe was always pretty, and I paid a lot of attention to my hair, shoes, and makeup—you'd never catch me without my false eyelashes! I wasn't threatening to my clients, and I did excellent work. But I felt like my size was holding me back from making it to the next level, which was my company's design team. The people on that team were a special class of usually very hip, fashionable-looking stylists. I didn't fit the part.

But I did so well at my salon that when I was ready for a change, they offered me a position in San Francisco. I couldn't wait for a fresh start in a new place!

SAN FRANCISCO

I really grew as an adult in San Francisco. My friends became my family—everyone in San Francisco is a transplant, so that's who your family becomes. And at work I was welcomed with open arms. I think I even lost weight! I was still chunky, but I felt the best I had felt in years. San Francisco is a city of nonjudgment. There was nothing for me to feel bad about. It was okay to have different opinions. You could disagree with someone and you'd still be friends the next day. I wasn't used to that kind of open-mindedness, and it was wonderful.

• •

STAY IN TOUCH

When you feel like you have nobody—you do. Make an effort to reach out for support, whether it's online or on the phone or by going to see a friend. Anything is possible, as long as you set up a support system you can tap into when you feel a bout of loneliness coming on.

• •

I had fallen in love, met the person who I felt was the love of my life. My partner was moving to Indonesia, and I had committed to making the move abroad, as well. I wasn't really sure I wanted to be in Indonesia, but I knew I wanted to be in the relationship.

We planned a huge going-away party—a luau in Golden Gate Park with a DJ and all of our friends. The day before the festivities, my grandmother called with devastating news: Grandpa had died. I completely broke down. Grandma told me to go ahead and have my party, and then fly home for the funeral. But when I got back to Arizona, I realized that my next move wasn't going to be to Indonesia. I decided to stay with my grandmother and help her through the transition of life without my grandfather. He had always taken care of her—she'd never paid a bill in her life; she'd never filled her own gas tank. I knew she needed my help. Within a week of Grandpa's funeral, I flew back to San Francisco, quit my job, packed my bags, and returned to Arizona for good.

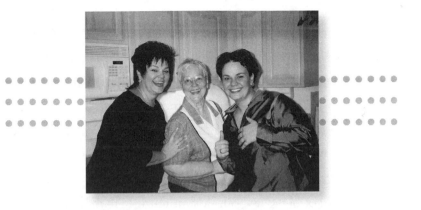

THREE

It Was My Destiny

I told the truth—how I wasn't happy where I was, I wasn't living the life that I wanted to live, I wasn't making the difference that I knew I could. And it wasn't easy to tell the truth about that.

I stayed with my grandma for about a year and a half. The first couple of months were great. I loved being able to help her, to take care of her. I took her to the store, filled up her car with gas.

Once I felt like she was okay, I moved out—and that's when I started to get really big.

I'd lost my grandpa, and in my transition back home, my relationship had ended with someone I'd loved. Even my dog, Sissy, the one constant in my life whom I adored, had unexpectedly died. I was devastated. It felt like I had given up on myself, my career, my dreams. I always thought I'd be a city girl and live in a place full of big ideas. But now, it felt like I would be stuck in Arizona forever. I didn't have a job, I'd gone through a lot of my savings, I didn't have a car. I started feeling empty—really empty. I ate and ate and never felt full. I'd been through so much in my life and had always managed to find some good in it. But this was desperately bad. Everything sucked. I was the biggest I'd ever been in my life—I had gained back the weight I'd lost in San Francisco, plus another 60 pounds or so. I was so far down a black hole, I didn't know how to get out.

I got a job at another salon and began working all the time, sometimes late into the night, if a client needed me. I ate fast food every day. I'd pick up breakfast from a drive-thru on the way to work. I probably drank three extra large lattes a day. I drank soda like it was going out of style. There was a candy dish at the salon, and I would grab a handful everytime I walked by. At night I would go out with my friends and drink at the bars—you couldn't put too much sugar on my lemon drop martinis. I wasn't eating regular meals; I just ate continuously all day.

My younger sister, Holly, had become a fan of *The Biggest Loser*, and she kept asking me to watch it with her. I hated the name—were they mocking fat people? I got angry when she would ask me—the "fat sister"—to watch. I know she was trying to help—my whole family was, because I'd told them I wanted to lose weight. Sometimes I'd go on bike rides with my stepmom, Peggy, and let her take "before" pictures of me. But my heart wasn't really in it—*they* wanted it more for me than *I* wanted it for me. I just kept thinking, "How did I get here? How did my life disappear, slip through my fingers?" I knew I was miserable, and miserable to be around.

My mom was thinking of getting gastric bypass surgery, and I considered it, too. But in the end I didn't want to do anything that I wasn't proud of. I felt that if I had surgery, it would mean that I hadn't done the real work, that I wasn't capable of controlling

· ·

DON'T BE A VICTIM

It wasn't easy to admit that maybe it was my fault that a relationship didn't work or that I wasn't promoted because of my attitude, not my image. It wasn't easy, but it was liberating. I realized that because a lot of times in my life I felt like the "victim," there was no room to change the situation. But once I dug deep and told the truth, I was able to acknowledge and forgive myself for the role I played in my pain and let go of it. I was carrying around years of hurt and feelings of being "less than," and I didn't need to. I realized that I was a strong woman, capable of creating her own destiny. I realized that I could choose.

· ·

myself, controlling my life. I know it's the right choice for some people. But it wasn't for me.

I finally saw a couple of episodes of *The Biggest Loser* and realized that it wasn't making fun of anyone—it was helping people get healthy. One night I was at my grandmother's house with my mom, who was sitting on the bed, eating hard candy and watching *The Biggest Loser*.

It was the finale episode of Season 3, when Eric Chopin won. I remember being mesmerized by the fact that this man had lost over 200 pounds. How the hell do you lose 200 pounds? How do you lose half your body weight? And it dawned on me: This show changes people's lives. I turned to Mom. I looked at her. I said, "I want to be on this show."

I've never seen her move so fast in her life. She flew out of bed, and the next thing I know, she's sitting at the computer, we're downloading an application, and I'm excited and scared and shaking . . . and having second thoughts. "Did I just say that? What am I talking about? I don't even watch TV. I don't have time to watch TV." I'm sitting on the floor, on my knees, and she's downloading the application. I freaked out. "Mom, stop," I said. "I'm not going to do it."

"What are you talking about? Of course you are!"

"No, I'm not. There's probably thousands of people doing this exact same thing at the exact same moment. They'd never choose me."

Because why would they?

• •

SET GOALS

One thing I realized when I got to *The Biggest Loser* ranch is that I'd stopped setting goals for myself. When you don't set goals, you deny yourself opportunities to succeed and celebrate. It's important to set realistic goals for yourself and rejoice when you achieve them.

• •

And so that was it. I stopped. She got back onto the bed. I left. I had seen the light and the possibility and thought, "I'm doing it!" I had felt my adrenaline rush, and my mom had flown off that bed, she was so excited for me. She wanted me to try something, anything, so I'd be happy again. She was tired of watching me beat myself up. She had been right there, and then it was over. I went back to my life again and tried to forget about it.

I GOT A TEXT MESSAGE

On a hot August night a few months later, I was working at the salon when I got a text message from my mom. It said, "Good news. BL's in town." I had no idea what she was talking about. What was "BL"? Some texting thing she'd just learned? (She had just started texting and using acronyms.) When I finished with my client, I called her.

"I just watched the weather forecast on the local news," she said, "and they said that *Biggest Loser* is doing an open casting call at the Mesa Arts Center on Saturday! You gotta go." Mom felt that if they just met me, they would choose me. In her mind, how could they not choose her Buba? "If you meet my Buba, you're going to fall in love with her," she thought. That's my mom. I'm her baby.

But I was fully booked on Saturday. I told her I wouldn't be able to make it.

"Mom, I can't afford to go," I said.

"Buba," Mom said, "you can't afford *not* to go."

I don't know what happened, but suddenly I said, "Okay, then you need to find out where I have to stand in line," and I hung up the phone. Then I called all my clients who had scheduled appointments for that day and told them that I had to reschedule.

The night before the auditions, I went out with my friends and partied away, got rip-roaring drunk. I was so scared. In the meantime, my mom and stepfather had ventured out to get the scoop on where the line for casting would form. When they found the location, the security guard told them that the producers were looking for *couples*. My mom said, "Oh, damn. I'm going to have

• •

SHARE YOUR DREAMS

Spread your excitement for change among your family and friends. Get them on board with your plans. That's how you can really bring about change in your life—by getting everyone to understand your dreams and goals and by asking for their support.

• •

to do this with her." Later Mom told me that she was the only fat person I knew, so she had to be my teammate. But that wasn't true. We both wanted to change our lives, and we didn't know anyone else who was ready for that kind of challenge. And besides—I wouldn't have wanted to do it with anyone else.

The next morning, I got up at 4:00 and put on my false eyelashes. I had been out so late the night before that I'd only slept for a few hours. But we were in line by 5:00 a.m., with no idea of what to expect. It just so happened that we were the 11th team in line. And it was August 11. So my mom walked up and down the line, telling everybody that they might as well go home, because they didn't stand a chance. The numbers were auspicious, she thought. We were given applications to fill out, and we realized we needed pictures. We didn't have any, so Mom ran to the nearest drugstore and bought a Polaroid camera while I kept our spot in line. When she got back, we took pictures of each other and fanned them in the air. We had no clue what we were doing, and Mom was embarrassing me, talking to every single person in line: "So, what's your story? Who are you here with? Oh, you're pretty!"

By 9:00 a.m., there were a few hundred people in line, and Mom knew everybody and everybody knew her, whether they wanted to or not. Some of these people had tried out for *Biggest Loser* before, and they had special outfits and routines that they were practicing. And there I was, tired, hungover, in my high heels and false eyelashes. The casting people finally began the process about an hour later. They had two big tables set up on the stage of an auditorium, and two groups of us would go up at a time. Mom and I were in the second group.

When it was our turn, we sat down at the table for our interview. This was our big chance. We had 10 minutes to make an impression. Everyone was trying to talk over everyone else because they wanted to be heard. It was overwhelming. My mom and I both shared a bit with the casting guy interviewing us—we liked him—but frankly, I don't even remember what I said. It was a lot to absorb.

But then we were taken to the back of the auditorium to fill out longer applications. Not everyone from our table was invited to the back—just us and the people in line that my mom had already identified as "cute" or "fun." I realized that we had just survived the first step in the process that could end up changing our lives. And I really, really wanted it.

OUT OF MY BODY WITH EXCITEMENT

All of us in that room were just so anxious and excited. . . and of course, having a good time. Because anywhere my mom is, there's a party.

A man came over to take our pictures, and Mom asked him if he could shoot us from above so that the angle would be more flattering. Of course, he was a skinny guy and probably never had to think about looking slimmer in a photo in his life. But Mom and I were cracking up, dropping down to the floor and posing to get below his lens. After they got the shots, we were sent home and told we'd get a phone call later in the week if the producers were interested in us.

We got a call that night.

I was out of my body with excitement. The following day we went to a hotel in Phoenix where the producers had reserved a suite for the next part of the casting process. We were videotaped for an hour and interviewed under those hot lights. I remember that I was wearing a knit shirt with three-quarter-length sleeves, because I wasn't comfortable with my arms. It was August in Arizona. Between the heat, the lights, and the nerves, I was sweating bullets. By the time the interview was over, my naturally curly hair—which I had straightened that morning—was curly again. Mom just stared at me, and I was so embarrassed. "Oh my heck," she said to the producers. "You guys don't understand. Buba must really want this, because I've never seen her so nervous."

I was so nervous that I don't remember much, but I do have one very clear memory: They asked us to pull up our shirts and show our stomachs. And that was really uncomfortable. I think I would have rather taken off my whole shirt than just shown my *belly*—which is what it was. My stomach had grown so huge that in my mind it was truly now a "belly."

I think once you make the decision to actually go stand in line at a *Biggest Loser* casting call, you know something has to change. I knew, after standing in that line and going through those interviews, that I was going to change my life regardless of whether I actually made it onto the show. And I knew that if I did make it to that ranch, it would be my biggest and best opportunity to do just that. I would be completely removed from my life, and I'd have an opportunity to tell the truth about a lot of things.

And I was ready. I was really ready. For a long time, I had been afraid of failing—but now I was tired of being afraid, tired of feeling like a loser. I wanted to become the Biggest Loser, the first female Biggest Loser!

OH MY GOSH, WE ARE GOING TO BE ON THIS SHOW

We got the call that the producers wanted us to be a part of the final interview process, which meant flying to Los Angeles and being sequestered in a hotel along with the other finalists. We had no way of knowing how long we'd be gone—it could be 3 days or almost 6 months. We weren't supposed to tell many people where we were going, so I just told my clients I'd be away for a while, and I'd be in touch when I got back.

We had to pack enough clothes for 6 months and were told that prints and black don't work on camera. I thought, "Do they have any idea what kind of clothes overweight women buy? My whole closet is prints and blacks!" Because that's all you can find in plus-size clothing. It's usually covered in loud print, or it's black.

When we got to our hotel room, we looked out our window and down at the pool. You could tell who the other hopeful contestants were from far away, because you'd see two big people being led around the pool by a tiny casting person. We stared down to examine our competition and invented their life stories—where they came from, who they were. There wasn't much else to do. We ended up being sequestered for a week.

We had more and more interviews and met with a nutritionist and a doctor. And in our downtime, we sat in our room having decadent "last suppers" of pizza and Mexican food and all the things we loved that we thought we'd probably never get to eat again. It's a familiar thought process for anyone who wants to lose weight: "I'm going to eat whatever I want until I start my diet." Back then, I didn't understand the thought process of healthy people, that you can eat the foods you want as long as you do so in moderation. But I didn't know anything about limits; I didn't know anything about budgeting calories. I used to eat so much in one sitting that I'd take breaks during my meals, I'd be so stuffed. I had to let it settle a little bit, but I wasn't done. I wanted to finish everything, but I had to take breathing breaks.

We still weren't 100 percent certain we were going to the ranch, but we went to wardrobe and were fitted in our spandex bra tops and bike shorts. All I could think was, "Oh my gosh, are we really going to be wearing this on national television?!"

Before I'd left, my brother-in-law, Andy (an avid *Biggest Loser* fan), had asked me, "So, if you make the show, are you going to go above or below?"

"Above or below?" I said. "What are you talking about? Above or below what?"

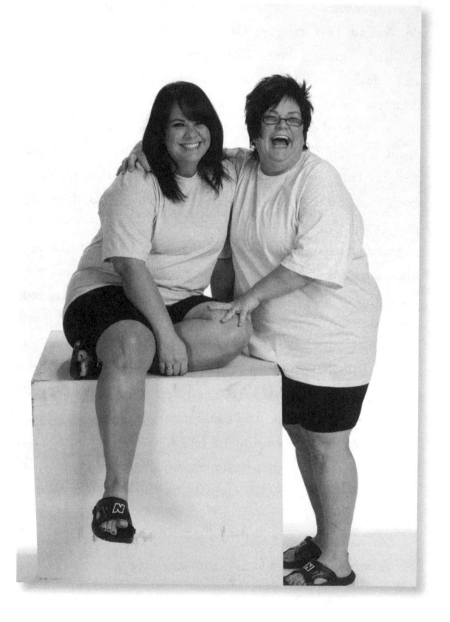

IT STARTS NOW

When I tried out for *The Biggest Loser,* I knew there was no turning back. I finally was going to do something, and I was going to do it for me, like you're doing it for you. I think it starts when you tell the truth that you're not happy with where you are in your life and admit you want to do something different. When you start your own journey, you have to constantly check in with yourself: Are you doing what you need to do for this process?

"You know, it's the big decision!" he answered. "Above or below the belly button?"

Well, I hadn't thought about that. It was funny, but he was right. If you look at all the contestants, the older women usually wear their shorts above the belly button, while the younger women wear them below.

I went with below.

ARE YOU KIDDING ME?

So at last it was time for the final interview with the NBC executives. The casting director told us, "This is it, you guys. If you're ever going to impress anybody, you have to impress these people." We were up first, and we were nervous. One of the executive producers was in the room. It was hard to see him because of all the bright lights and people milling around in the background. We were being filmed, the lights were shining on us. They asked us more questions.

The second time we went back to that room, we were joined by another group of potential contestants. And then the executive announced to all of us, "I want you to remember how you're feeling in this moment." We had all made it onto the show! We started cheering and crying; so much emotion was coming out of everyone. He told us to always remember how excited we were because this was the moment when our lives started to change. He said that soon we'd start referring to our lives as "before" *The Biggest Loser* and "after" *The Biggest Loser* because difficult times were ahead.

I couldn't get that idea out of my mind. Even though I knew I wanted to be the first female Biggest Loser, I thought there was no way a TV show or any experience like it would become such a defining moment in my life. I had been saying that I wanted it, and I knew that I did, but I didn't think it would compare to other big changes I'd experienced. I'd led a pretty interesting life, filled with lots of big moments. I'd been an internationally ranked athlete. I had gone through difficult things. I'd lost people I loved.

When we returned to our room, the cupcakes Mom and I had bought earlier in anticipation of just such a celebration were sitting on a table, waiting for us. We put them in a bag and called the front desk to see if someone could come up and take them out of our room.

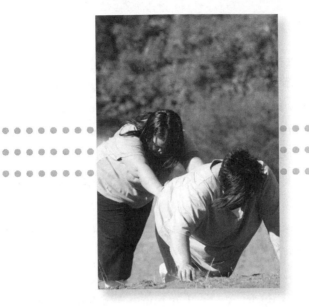

FOUR

Scared Every Second

*I just took the bull by the horns, and I was
scared. I was scared every second of every day.*

All the contestants were driven out to King Gillette
Ranch, about 45 minutes outside Los Angeles. We
still weren't allowed to talk to the other teams—the
producers wanted to catch our initial reactions to
one another and the conversations on camera. When our van
pulled up to the security desk at the front gate of the campus, we
were told to get out and stretch.

Then the production team began to film us each walking onto the ranch with our teammate, in pairs. One of the producers shouted, "Back to one!" and we had to retrace our steps and do it all over again. "Back to one" is a phrase we got to know really well on the ranch. It's production talk for repositioning the cameras so that they can get a better shot. That day, there was a lot of "Back to one"—Mom and I ended up doing the walk onto the ranch so many times that we were exhausted before we even made it to where host Alison Sweeney was standing! Just walking to our first challenge was tiring for us at that point. We had no idea how much harder it was about to get.

Alison explained that our first challenge involved choosing our trainers. Each team had to hike up the mountain on campus and then come all the way back to where we started. Trainers Bob

• •

USE YOUR BODY WEIGHT

One of the biggest realizations I had on the ranch is that using the resistance of your own body weight is enough to get results. We used a lot of very basic exercises—the stuff I learned as a kid in gym class, like squats, lunges, jumping jacks, pullups, and push-ups. Don't get me wrong—I am a huge advocate of working out in a gym. But I love knowing that if there's no gym in sight, I still have control over my workouts and my physical health.

• •

Harper and Jillian Michaels would be waiting for us at the finish line, and the teams that crossed in the fastest times could pick their trainer. Those who finished last wouldn't have a choice. Mom and I decided that we needed someone incredibly tough to push us.

We wanted Jillian.

If you happened to watch that first episode, you saw for yourself that I literally had to push my mom on her butt up to the top of the mountain. She was completely out of breath and exhausted. She could barely walk. She was so thirsty, and there was no water. At one point I asked her if she wanted me to spit in her mouth (she said no, thankfully)—it was that bad. In a way, I was grateful that I seemed to have more stamina than she did, because I wasn't sure if I was going to make it. I had no choice but to keep going and to help my mom. I kept thinking, "What in the world have we gotten ourselves into?" Mom was exhausted, and she said she wanted to quit. I got really upset with her.

"What's the point, Buba?" she said.

"What's the point?! The point is that we finish!" I answered.

We finished that race dead last. And what you didn't get to see on the show is just *how much* later we crossed the finish line than the team before us. We were probably in last place by an hour, but they obviously had to trim the long wait for TV. It was our first challenge, and Mom and I were already on an emotional roller coaster. I was mad at her because she didn't want to finish;

she already wanted to quit when we had just started.

By the time we got to the finish line, Jillian's team had filled up, so we ended up with Bob as our trainer. And we were upset about that. We just felt Jillian would be the one to kick our butts into shape. When Bob handed out the T-shirts for his team, Mom and I got pink ones. The funny thing is, now I think of pink as my signature color—but at the time, I wasn't thrilled. In competitive swimming, a pink ribbon is not so great—it's like eighth place. And eighth place just wasn't going to cut it for me.

ON AND OFF CAMERA

We were working really hard to lose weight at the ranch, of course, but we were also being filmed for a television show—so there was a whole production schedule that we had to fit into our days, in addition to all of our workouts. Even on "rest days" (our one day off from the gym each week), we still had to do interviews on camera. In fact, when I got home from the ranch, I actually found it easier to fit in all my workouts, because my time wasn't consumed by interviews!

I get questions all the time about what was it like to live on the ranch in front of the cameras. Weird, at first, as you might imagine. You're steaming broccoli in the kitchen and the camera guys are right there filming it. You're sitting down at the table to eat your broccoli and the cameras are filming that. It's what they call in the TV world, "reality." Those were times on the ranch when nothing special was planned, but we had to make ourselves available in the kitchen or living room, for example, to have our interactions filmed. We'd often just sit around and talk, sometimes I'd cut someone's hair. But I couldn't do anything drastic—for show continuity, they don't like the contestants to drastically alter the appearance of their hair in the early stages of the show.

Brittany played a trick on the crew one time by covering up her long dark hair with a short wig cut into a bob. A producer flew into the room to ask if I had cut her hair! My mom was there and said that her Buba would never cut that bad of a bob.

After a while, you just get used to it. Everyday, you lose a little bit more of your reserve. I got used to just holding out my arm and letting someone put a mike up my bra! I got used to three people touching me at the same time. Toward the end, if I was wearing a sweaty T-shirt on camera and they wanted me to change into something fresh, I could just pull that t-shirt off right then and there (sports bra on, of course) and pull on a new one. Ok, ready? Action! You can't be modest and be on a reality TV show.

There are cameras manned by camera people and there are cameras and microphones planted all over the ranch to catch contestant action. We made a game out of looking for them. Were they in that plant? Was there a mic behind that picture? We knew there were cameras in our bedrooms, you could see them mounted right up in the corners. Sometimes Mark, for example, would get fed up and toss a towel over his bedroom camera. Minutes later there would be a gentle knock on the door. "Um, Mark? Can you take the towel off the camera?" It would be a production assistant dispatched from the control room next to the gym, where all the TV monitors are watched and conversations listened to day and night by a note-taking production crew. Believe me, if something interesting starts to happen, they're going to consider developing it or weaving it into a story line.

The only sacred spot, guaranteed to be camera-free, was your bathroom. But even there, if two or more people were gathered, you had to expect to be visited by a camera crew! You got used to cameras in your face when you were sweating and dying on the treadmill. I would just focus on something in the distance to not be distracted by a cameraman lying on his back below me, getting his shot.

We had microphones placed on our bodies everyday except for rest days. We'd be given a call sheet each night for the next day and told what time we had to be downstairs for getting our microphones placed. Outside of our group activities, we had individual interviews with producers almost everyday. The thing is, you don't know what others are saying in their interviews, so it's really interesting to see what others were thinking, if it makes it on the show when the season airs. You don't know what the trainers are saying on camera, for example. There's an element of surprise for everyone.

Sometimes when we had to travel by van for the challenges, we needed to get up really early in the morning in order to arrive at the location of the shoot and have good light. Other times, we'd do a challenge at night and drive back really late. When you're already changing the habits your body is used to, getting up extra early or staying up extra late can add even more stress. I decided to take advantage of every minute I had, so I would bring my pillow and a sleeping mask with me in the van to catch a few more hours of sleep. I'd get in a quick nap anytime I could. It gave me a chance to rest, and when the other contestants were too tired to exercise, I was still able to do another workout. Sometimes I'd bring my jump rope with me, too, so I could get in a little workout while we waited for the shoot to start.

In the beginning, I definitely bonded with Jenni Westphal. We were in similar situations—our partners were our parents. Jenni really struggled with her dad, Lynn, making it to the gym and doing the physical challenges. And my mom was exhausted and tired a lot. Jenni and I were on the same team, and we related to each other's struggles.

LEARNING HOW TO EAT

When we first arrived at the ranch, Bob talked to us about our calorie budgets and what we needed to eat—mainly veggies, fruit, protein, whole grains, and low-fat dairy—something we had also learned from our consultations with the show's nutritionist, Cheryl Forberg, RD. But it was so much information to take in at once, I just felt lost in the beginning. I took notes and looked back at them frequently. I began to grasp the principles of healthy eating over time, but it took concentration and hard work.

On our rest days, we were allowed to eat a few more calories than on normal days. It wasn't a binge day or a cheat day, but a higher-calorie day that we had to plan for, and that Bob had to approve in advance. We were allowed to eat treats like a slice of pizza or a burger, and that's how I began to understand that once I left the ranch, I'd be able to incorporate my favorite foods into my long-term weight loss goals. It's all about planning. And of course, the next day, we went right back to our regular fitness and eating routine.

Before I arrived on campus, I didn't cook—I nuked. And, contrary to what viewers probably think, there are no chefs on *The Biggest Loser* ranch. It's a strictly do-it-yourself operation when it comes to cooking. The few things I did know how to make were fattening dishes like pasta with creamy sauce or Mexican food smothered in cheese. But the kitchen at the ranch is a pretty impressive place. There are cabinets brimming with spices and seasonings, refrigerators stocked with fresh fruit and vegetables, and freezers full of healthy proteins like chicken and fish. We didn't have to worry about grocery shopping—it was all there for us. But if you really liked a particular fruit or vegetable, you had to make sure you chopped it up and stored it in a plastic bag with your name on it so no one else would eat it!

There are also stacks of *Biggest Loser* cookbooks everywhere with tons of healthy recipe ideas. Most days I was so tired, I just made really simple foods. Mom was exhausted from the very beginning, and I don't think she would have eaten if I hadn't cooked for her and brought meals to our room. She could barely get out of bed

SNACKING WITH YOUR FAMILY

Make sure you always have your own low-calorie snacks on hand so that if your family sits down for a bowl of ice cream, for example, you've got your nonfat Greek yogurt with berries or your low-fat frozen yogurt. You can't always ask your family to eradicate ice cream from the freezer, but you can be proactive about having what you need readily available.

those first few weeks. Roger Shultz and Trent Patterson were equally perplexed by the kitchen, so when I made meals for Mom and me, I'd throw some extra chicken, squash, peppers, onions, and mushrooms into the sauté pan for them as well.

The hardest part was learning to weigh and measure every ingredient. But I had to know how many calories I was eating, so I'd measure out a cup or half cup of each ingredient for each person eating the dish so I'd know how many calories were in each portion. I learned to become aware of what a portion size should look like and how much food was going into my body. I became very detail oriented. I didn't want to leave anything to chance!

I was eating vegetables like never before. I really didn't like them at first, but I knew I needed to change my eating habits, and there was such a nice selection of fresh vegetables at the ranch. I added tomato salsa to a lot of my meals, which gave them the spicy flavor I loved with hardly any added calories. I'd had spaghetti squash before and showed everyone else at the ranch how to cook them. One night I made spaghetti squash topped with a sauce of ground turkey and veggies, like a regular pasta dish. Everyone loved it! It was fun to try out new things and cook healthier versions of the foods we used to eat.

The funny thing is, when you stop eating junk and start eating healthy food, you begin to acquire a taste for it more than the junk. I never used to eat tomatoes, for example, and at the ranch I was eating them all the time. And onions and garlic—I hated them before, but now I love them on everything.

In the beginning, I wasn't that hungry. But as I got leaner and healthier, my appetite really revved up. Jillian said that was good because my metabolism had really kicked in. We'd all gotten our metabolisms working full-bore again because of the exercise we were doing. We wore Bodybuggs—armband monitors that track your calories consumed and burned. I lived and died by the numbers on that Bodybugg. We logged our food and workouts so that we could see how many calories we burned and what our deficit was each day. Once I knew I had burned enough calories, then I could sleep!

WORKING OUT AT THE RANCH

As the weeks went on, the workouts didn't get any easier. Or at least, they never felt easier. Bob and Jillian are the best at what they do, and they constantly pushed us. On our second week at the ranch, Bob and Jillian decided to try doing things a little differently than in past seasons, and they co-trained all of us, abandoning the team concept for a while. Mom and I actually ended up training a lot with Jillian. She knew her stuff and really watched people's results. We felt like she was as committed to helping us change our lives as we were. I appreciated her intensity.

Every contestant on *The Biggest Loser* comes to the ranch thinking the workouts are going to start gradually. They don't. Even that first day, from that first challenge, we were exhausted. There was not one single day on the ranch when I wasn't sore. But I knew I would finish the workout. It was like being in that glass factory back in Texas. I just had to do one thing at a time. If I could do it once, I could do it again. So I just got used to the soreness. I was learning to live outside of my comfort zone, which in turn was teaching me how to grow up.

• •

DON'T GET IN A WORKOUT RUT

One thing I learned from Jillian is that you always have to mix up your workout routines. Try everything. I spin, swim, kickbox, lift weights. There's not one thing I won't try that's physical. I think that's how I was able to not only lose weight but create a strong, toned body.

• •

We basically spent 6 to 8 hours a day working out—sometimes 10 hours, toward the end. We were usually trained by Bob and Jillian for about 4 hours, and the rest of the time we did our "homework"—workouts we had to do on our own, like putting in a few hours on the stairclimber or elliptical, doing a certain number of reps with weights. Our homework was usually done at a more moderate pace than the training, which was intense and focused. The only breaks we had were to use the bathroom (there was a little portable bathroom outside the gym) or to refill our water bottles. And Jillian always kept an eye on how long we were gone. You could only have so many bathroom breaks!

Occasionally a producer would interrupt a training session and grab one of us for an interview, and I used to pray that I would get picked so I could take a break. Even then, sometimes Jillian wouldn't let us go—she'd tell the producer we couldn't leave until we finished our workout.

There's also a pool at the ranch, though I was the only one who ever really swam. It was cold at first; then they started heating it. I got to know the pool maintenance guy who came to clean it, because I was always waiting for him to come. He said he was happy someone was using it.

TIME FOR CONFESSIONAL

When you watch the show, and see a contestant talking straight to the camera alone in a room, you know they're in the "confessional." Upstairs, above the kitchen, on the same floor where the bedrooms are, is a room filled with camera equipment and a stool. We were taught how to turn on the camera so we could go into the room anytime and just start talking to camera alone. You can pour your heart out or just review your day, which is usually what I did. I was very focused on losing weight and generally avoided politics, so I don't know if I was that interesting in confessional! The only time I really let fly was late in the season when I felt like the guys ganged up on Kelly and me. I was so offended by how the guys acted in that challenge, not even giving us a chance.

The funny thing about the confessional room is that even though it seems like you're alone, you're not! If the camera is out of focus while you're talking, you'll hear a phone ring. You pick it up and someone asks, "Ali, can you sit a little more to the right?" If a day goes by and you haven't gone to confessional, you'll get a gentle knock on your door, asking you to go to please do so. The truth is, you definitely have a job as a contestant—not only are you putting in the workout hours, you have to put in the production hours as well.

THE FIRST WEIGH-IN

Weigh-in days were always tense. If there were alliances in play, people were nervous about whether they'd be supported or sold out by their friends. Mom and I never relied on alliances. We just tried to be supportive and friendly to everyone. I never wanted to get rid of anyone. I just wanted to lose as much weight as I could each week to stay above the dreaded "yellow line." If your weekly

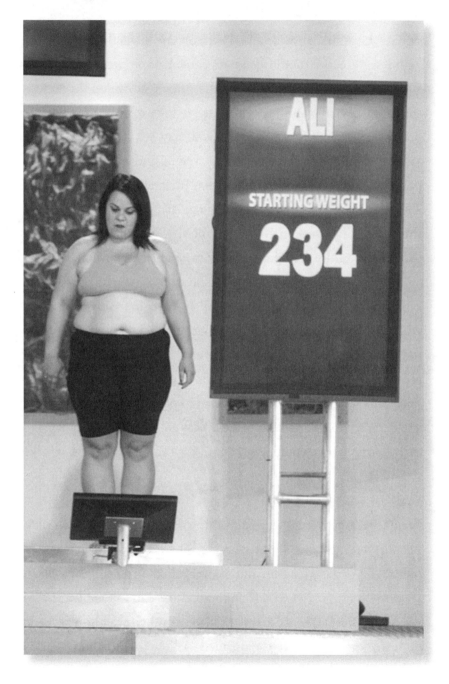

percentage of weight loss wasn't high enough, you fell below the yellow line, making you eligible for elimination.

The day of a weigh-in was usually quiet, with no scheduled workouts, and I wanted every second I could have to rest. It was the only day of the week I put on makeup to try to look nice on camera. The weigh-in process itself lasted 3 hours or so, through the various takes. It was excruciating to stand there for so long.

After a week on the ranch, it was time for our first weigh-in. Before it began, one of the contestants passed around a piece of paper and asked everyone to write down their e-mail addresses and phone numbers so that we could keep in touch after being sent home. I wouldn't add my information. I was not going to risk submitting to the possibility that we would be eliminated.

I also knew that some of the contestants didn't like my mom's personality and that if we fell below the yellow line, we'd probably be sent home. And that made me furious. So what if she was loud and outspoken? It was her way of dealing with stuff she was going through, all the pain and the struggle. Just getting out of bed every morning of that first week was difficult; I knew she literally had to crawl out because her body hurt so much. And then it was off to the gym for another workout! I remember lying on the bed one morning and looking at her, wondering if she would be okay. I knew she had to do this to save her life, but I didn't know if it was going to kill her in the process. So for anyone else not to respect her drive and have some compassion for her struggle made me mad. We were all going through the same process.

• •

Don't Worry about What Others Think

All you can control is what you put into your body and what you burn off your body. As my body started to get stronger every day at *The Biggest Loser* ranch, I began to realize that I didn't need to worry about who was in an alliance with whom. I just needed to remember that I could do whatever I put my mind to.

• •

I was literally scared to tears waiting to climb up on that giant scale. As the weigh-in progressed, all the teams with male team members posted huge numbers—the guys were dropping weight fast. Mom and I, along with Jenn Widder and Maggie King, were the only two all-female teams, and women don't typically lose weight as quickly as men do. So I was terrified that we were all going to fall below the yellow line.

The first weigh-in seemed to go on forever, and as I watched all those impressive numbers come up on the scale, I thought, "There's no way we can do this, just no way. And I don't want to go home—I need this. I want this." And then I just burst, I literally burst, into tears and started bawling. Everyone stared at me, wondering what was going on. I just couldn't take the pressure anymore.

But the next thing I knew, it was our turn, and we walked up to the scale. The numbers came up on the screen, and Mom had lost 16 pounds, and I'd lost 19! We came in second for the highest percentage of weight loss that week. It felt amazing. It felt redemptive.

When I was on the ranch, we had an hour to deliberate after the weigh-in finished, before we met again for the elimination. That first week's elimination went pretty smoothly. The two teams to fall below the yellow line were the father-daughter team of Lynn and Jenni Westphal and the best friends team of Maggie King and Jenn Widder. As I've said, I was close to Jenni as someone who also had a middle-aged parent as a teammate, but Lynn was pretty clear with us that he felt he didn't need to be on the ranch to lose the weight. We were all so grateful for our time on the ranch that if someone expressed indifference to being there, it made our elimination decision much easier.

LETTING GO OF OLD HURTS

Being on the ranch with my mom was such a delicate yet amazing experience. At that point, she was the oldest woman ever to be on campus, and she was really proud of that. But I know it was hard for her to feel like one of the weaker links. In my family, we didn't do things unless we thought we could win. We focused on a sport we were good at and then excelled at it. I focused on swimming, even though I'd always wanted to play volleyball or softball growing up. But I didn't know if I could be good at them, and my sister and I weren't encouraged to play other sports. For both my mom and me, learning new things—some of which we weren't the best at—was challenging. I was never a consistently strong competitor at the challenges, but I started to realize that that was part of the journey.

As we trained more and more with Jillian, I knew she was starting to sniff out our unique mother-daughter dynamic. Jillian was all about separating teammates as much as possible, especially those who came to the ranch with major enabling mechanisms in place. Her first big move in separating my mom and me came when we were working out in the gym one day and my mom fell off the treadmill next to me. I immediately jumped off my treadmill to help her, and Jillian screamed at me.

"No!" she said. "You guys are separate. You don't get to police each other anymore or save each other anymore. Quit mothering your mom."

Rescuing my mom was not the answer to my problems—or hers. I knew that I tried to protect my mother. On the one hand, I resented that she hadn't been around as much as I wanted her to be when I was a kid. I had so wanted a normal, stable childhood without all the chaos Amber and I were subjected to. I hated some of the situations she put us in, living with different boyfriends, falling asleep in a chair at parties after having too much to drink, getting furious at me for being friendly with my stepmom. On the other hand, I loved her. She was my mom. And I defended her whenever I felt she was being criticized. I didn't think anyone had the right to attack her.

Our fights over the years were often triggered when I felt she was judging me for how I was living my life. I wanted her to understand that some of my lifestyle choices were a reflection of

● ●

WHO COMES FIRST?

One thing I learned from being on the ranch with my mom was that I had to change myself first. That's the only way I could then accept support from and offer support to her. Letting go of trying to take care of her helped me get my emotional balance back. It's probably one of the most challenging parts of weight loss: knowing that in order to truly give to others, you have to give to yourself first.

● ●

what I'd learned from her—like partying too much or not valuing myself enough and making bad decisions. Other times, I just tried to express the pain of my childhood to her, of feeling so lonely and abandoned. But she would get defensive and tell me she was not the cause of my misery.

Jillian had asked me, point-blank, if I thought I could keep the weight off without addressing these painful memories with Mom. And deep down, I knew I couldn't, though I dreaded the idea of confronting her about it. I knew that if I didn't dig through this situation, I wouldn't come out on the other side. I couldn't change by holding on to so much hurt.

Finally, during our third week at the ranch, after another exhausting workout, I was in the kitchen getting a snack. Jillian came in and said she wanted me to go out to what we call the prison yard, a big patio area off the kitchen where we sometimes did outdoor workouts. I had no idea that the time had come. But as she led me out, I saw Mom, sitting there, leaning up against a wall, looking as exhausted and spent as I'd ever seen her look. I felt like I had walked into a minefield.

"No, I'm not doing this," I said.

"You have to do it," Jillian said.

With Jillian standing there, I told Mom how alone I had felt growing up. I told her that I didn't want to be unhappy anymore, I didn't want to be in this body anymore, and I was tired of being stuck. I admitted that the weight was a result of more than just eating too much.

Mom was, frankly, amazing. Her defenses were down. She told me that she knew she had brought a lot of "riffraff" around when I was young, that she had stayed out too much, and that she was sorry for that. She said she never wanted me to feel alone, she wanted to be there for me from now on. She acknowledged that she had had two kids who'd raised her, and that she wasn't proud of that. "I love you more than life," she said. "Why do you think I came to this dumb old place? I wanted to be with *you*."

It was a huge moment for us. That moment was the only time we talked about our issues on the ranch, but it was all I needed. Being on *The Biggest Loser* was probably the first truly unconditional motherly thing that I knew with all my heart she did for me. I know my mother only went on that campus for me. It was all about her Buba.

The experience of being on *The Biggest Loser* ranch bares your soul. There's no hiding. You are completely vulnerable. Everywhere I go, people want to hear my weight loss story. But my weight loss story is part of the journey of my life, a journey toward accepting myself just the way I am and loving myself just the way I am. Of course the physical part is important—tracking calories, burning calories, eating right, all that stuff. But for me at least, that's about 10 percent of the equation. That's just a matter of doing. Facing my emotions and letting myself separate from my mom were much harder than any physical challenge. For the first time in my life, I was giving myself a break.

THE LETTERS

By week 4, all of us had finally started to feel like we would be able to physically survive this experience. We had gotten used to the pain.

Paul Marks and Kelly Fields really pushed themselves that week, and they won the challenge. The reward for this was being able to read letters from our loved ones. Even though Paul and Kelly had won, they decided to let all of us, their opponents, get the letters instead.

I remember thinking that getting a letter from home wasn't such a big deal. Great for people who had kids or spouses, I thought, but not for me. Looking back on it, I think I had drifted away and secluded myself so much over the years that I didn't really feel close to my family. To be honest, I don't think I expected anybody to send me a letter.

As it turned out, I got letters from my grandma; my sister, Amber;

my dad; my stepmom; and all my other siblings. Amber and I had always stuck together, through all the tough times in our childhood. Even when Amber wanted to move in with our dad and I didn't want to, I did it anyway because I felt we belonged together. We were like opposite halves of the same person—I was the messy tomboy, and she was neat and organized. But I also took advantage of her sometimes. As a teenager, I would grab things out of her closet that I liked and never return them. And as an adult, I would borrow money from her, and she would wipe the slate clean every Christmas.

When she eventually got married, it was hard for me. I felt as if she'd left me. Amber moved to Spokane, Washington, to be with her husband. I always judged her marriage and criticized her choices. I didn't like the way she was living her life, and I let her know how I felt.

Sitting next to my mom in our room at the ranch, I opened up my letter from Amber and read it out loud for the whole world to hear:

Dear Ali,

I am your biggest fan and you're my little sister who's always taken care of me. You are a natural leader, and it's only natural that you would lead Mom to and through this. You are so loving and one of the most giving people I know. I am so proud to be your sister. You were there for me and everyone else but now it's time for you to be that person for yourself. Somewhere along the line I think you

*decided that you didn't deserve it, and I'm here to tell you
that you do. You deserve it all and more, and I am cheering
for you every day. You are worth it. Keep it up.*
All my love,
Amber

Mom was in tears, and I was in tears as I finished reading it.
I felt so bad that I had cut off communication and let myself
become isolated from everyone who loved me and wanted to help.
My entire life, Amber had been there for me. But over the years,
I had not allowed her to support me, because the truth is, she
could call me on my stuff, and I didn't want to be called out. So
I stopped reaching out to her. I realized that she had always been
my biggest fan—I'd just forgotten.

I finished reading through the rest of the letters, and at the
end, I was just dumbfounded. My family believed in me. I just
hadn't believed in myself.

GAME OVER

That week I dropped 8 pounds and fell below the 200 mark. And
I thought, "Never again." Football players weigh over 200 pounds!
For my height, 5 feet 5 inches, it's not acceptable. My progress
was great, but we were still competitors in a game. And the game
was about to take over.

Mark and Jay Kruger were the week's Biggest Losers, which
meant they would have immunity at the elimination. And Paul

and Kelly, whom Mom and I had voted to send home the previous week, beat all of us. So they would choose who went home. Mom and I were not in a good position.

In the elimination room, Paul and Kelly decided to send us home. I couldn't believe it was happening. I had known in my heart that I was going to be the first female Biggest Loser, I had worked hard, I had proven I could do this—and now I was heading home? I was afraid I wasn't going to be able to keep up my healthy new lifestyle at home. I was not ready to deal with my life back in Arizona, but I was still determined. I told everyone in that elimination room that I would eventually be the Biggest Loser. Something inside would not let me give up that easily.

We had packed our bags before the elimination, and they were already in the van waiting for us as we walked out of the elimination room. I had to find strength. I kept thinking, "I'm going to do this. I'm going to show up at that finale with the highest percentage of weight loss. Someone else will have the title, but everyone will know that I won, that it was possible for a woman to do it, for *me* to do it."

We left the ranch and got to our hotel at around 2:00 or 3:00 in the morning. And then at 7:00 the next morning, we were taken to the airport. And that was it. I was sitting on that airplane, and I was going home. It was over. Now what? Some friends showed up to greet us when we landed at the Phoenix airport, and I was happy to see them, but I needed some time for myself. I was still going to be the first female Biggest Loser, one way or another. I just had to figure out how I was going to get there.

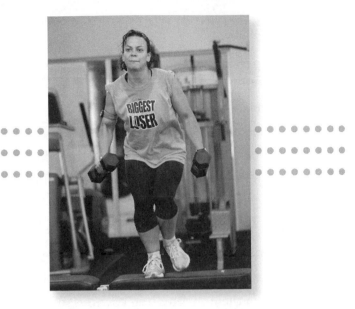

FIVE

I Got a Phone Call

This time I owned it, to my very core.

That first night back home, I was overwhelmed. I just wasn't ready. I wasn't ready to see anybody. I wasn't ready to talk about anything. I was a different person, but I didn't know how to communicate that. So this is what I did: I immediately went back to the old Ali—for one night. I went out with my friends, hit the town, and stayed out all night partying. I woke up hungover the next day and thought, "What in the hell? You can't do this. This is not who you are anymore. This is not worth the rest of your life."

I was on the verge of changing my life, of growing up, but now I was right back in the same environment where the old Ali had been so stuck and so unhappy. And I was feeling vulnerable. I needed to find a safe haven to make sure my new healthy habits didn't dissolve. I needed to keep reinforcing my new lifestyle over and over and in a place where I wasn't constantly put to the test. I knew how to make the right choices, but I didn't always have the strength to make them in tempting circumstances. So I decided to literally childproof my life.

AN OFFER OF LOVE

My younger sister Holly was pregnant. She and her husband, Andy, lived in Chandler, Arizona, a few towns over from me.

• •

GRAB HOLD

The best way to deal with a setback is to just really grab hold. Reach out to your friends and family and ask for their support. Make sure your home doesn't harbor temptations, and go to the gym immediately. Tell everyone if they want to find you, you'll be at the gym! Do whatever it takes, but take told of that tailspin. Tailspins will happen. It's just a matter of how you deal with them and take control of the situation.

• •

Andy called me and said, "Look, you've done so well, and we want you to be able to have the support you need and not have to worry about anything. We want you to be around people who care about you and your goals. I'm inspired by what you've accomplished so far, and I just think it would be really good if you could come live with us and help Holly out and show me how to eat and work out. You could help me, too."

It was an incredibly generous, loving offer. I wasn't sure about accepting it at first. I had gotten so used to taking care of myself and doing everything on my own. But everyone knew the house I was living in with my roommates was a party house. And I needed to remove myself from situations that weren't going to be able to change with me. I needed the help and support of my sister and brother-in-law—I didn't want to do this alone. And I loved that Andy thought that I could help them, too, and him in particular.

I talked to my roommates and told them that as much as I loved them, I couldn't stay in the house anymore. It was really hard, because they were my close friends, and it felt like I was abandoning them. But I just couldn't live in such a crazy environment anymore. I had to have the energy to wake up and go work out—before and after work—so I knew I had to change my schedule and change my lifestyle, and it wasn't their fault. I was choosing this, and I didn't think they needed to pay the price for my choices, so I had to go.

It was tough to leave the security of my friends and the life I was used to, but I knew I had to take care of me—and I needed to feel okay about that. I needed to understand that taking care of me wasn't selfish. It was what was best for me.

People started coming out of the woodwork to help me, especially my family. I got some personal training from my brother Joey, who played football and knows a ton of drills. He had a full-time job and a new home to take care of, but he made time in his schedule to help me stay on track. It also became a great way for me to bond with him. Joey made my workouts fun by taking them out of the gym. We'd go to the park and do step drills on the curbs and throw weighted balls up in the air. I was crawling, I was rolling—and I was laughing! He had all the coach's equipment: a whistle and a stopwatch. He was as serious about my workouts as I was!

FAMILY ON BOARD

My dad's family wanted to go to Mexico for a traditional family Christmas, which I knew would involve celebrating with lots of extra calories—eating Mexican food, drinking alcohol, sampling desserts. It wasn't really the kind of situation that felt safe for me to be in. I didn't want to stay behind over the holidays, but it looked like I would have to, for the sake of my goals. But here's what happened: My family wanted me to go with them so much that they created menus with healthy choices and offered to split up cooking duties every day so that I could eat with them and have fun, too.

There wasn't a gym in our house in Mexico, so my brothers all helped me work out while we were away. We found a little basketball court, and I did drills there with anything I could push, pull, or carry. We used jump ropes and had pushup challenges. We ran up and down sand dunes on the beach and hiked with weights. Sometimes that weight was my niece Avery, Holly's daughter. She was about a year and a half old and a nice, big, healthy girl! I carried her on my back. I let my Bodybugg tell me when I could stop. One day I had 30 calories left to burn according to my Bodybugg, so I wouldn't let myself sit down and play cards with everyone until I was satisfied that they were gone. My younger brother Adam and I, laughing our heads off, just shimmied on the back patio until those calories had vanished. That was my exercise *aha!* moment. I realized you don't have to always be on the treadmill or in step class to burn calories. You can just do whatever moves you in the moment. You can just be joyfully active!

For Christmas presents, we exchanged gifts that promoted

• •

FITNESS ON THE ROAD

I travel with a jump rope just in case I have no other option for working out. I guess the bottom line is where there's a will, there's a way. No matter what, you have choices. Travel with a workout video or stretch bands, or take a walk in your hotel parking lot. But be creative.

• •

health—heart rate monitors, workout equipment, things like that. It was one of the best Christmases I'd ever spent with my family. That Christmas was all about supporting me, and who could ask for a more generous and loving gift than that?

GETTING IT TOGETHER

At Holly's house, we cleaned out the refrigerator and pantry and bought all the stuff I had been eating at the ranch: fresh fruits and veggies, lean meats, whole grain carbs, and low-fat dairy. I cooked meals for us, showing Holly and Andy how to weigh and measure every ingredient and how to get flavor from herbs and spices, not added fats. And I introduced them to my favorite spaghetti squash recipe!

I focused on fueling my body. I ate within half an hour of waking up every morning: oatmeal and some fruit, or half of an Ezekiel muffin with an egg over easy and a slice of turkey bacon. Then I would eat every 3 to 4 hours after that. I would veggie-load my meals, because vegetables provided bulk and not many calories, and they made me feel full.

I went back to salon work and had more clients, but I also scheduled times to eat during the workday. I had to retrain myself and the people around me. When I was in the back room eating a meal or snack, I did not jump up to handle a walk-in client. I was eating. I was refueling my body. I was taking care of myself. And that time was sacred. I would not be disturbed.

I negotiated for a lower training fee at my gym. I still had bills to pay, and I wasn't working a full schedule at the salon. I started waking up early in the morning to go on bike rides with Peggy. Then I would head to the gym. I really tried to be a morning person in the beginning, pushing myself to get in a lot of exercise before a certain time. For some reason, I always thought that healthy people got up early—so I needed to do that, too, right? But I was trying to change everything about myself at once— my living situation, my meals, my sleeping schedule, my working schedule. I was burning the candle at both ends. One day, my dad sat me down and said, "Ali, you're making a lot of changes right now. But you're not a morning person. Just be okay with that."

He was right—it was too much. So I learned to relax a bit and let my day start a little later.

I learned to listen to my body and understand when it needed rest. If you're too tired, you're not going to get the most out of your workout anyway, and it's going to take longer to achieve results, because you can't perform at a high level. Getting enough sleep can be just as important as working out.

I arranged my schedule so that I had 2 days off in the week for rest and recuperation. But the other days were really intensive workout days. In addition to my bike rides and working out at the gym, I got my mom to join me, because she was feeling lost. She would come to my gym in the morning, and we'd do fun stuff like boxing or plyometric drills (for power training). Sometimes we'd play soccer or jump rope. Then I would usually have lunch, and Mom would go home and go for a walk. After lunch, I'd take a nap so that I could go back to the gym that night to work out with my brother.

I didn't count the hours of working out. Again, I just watched my Bodybugg, and when it told me I had burned the number of calories I needed to burn that day, I rested. I find that if you have some way of tracking your calories, then weight loss and maintenance becomes a mathematical equation—calories in and calories out. It's liberating.

I was putting into practice everything I'd learned at *The Biggest Loser* ranch. And it was working.

GETTING BACK IN TOUCH

After being at my sister's house for a while and getting into a routine, I started to really miss my friends. Maintaining friend-

• •

NIGHT EATING

I know there's advice out there about not eating after a certain time at night or eating very lightly at night. I don't really think about it that way. I think about what I'm going to be doing after I eat. I try to think of food as fuel. If I'm going straight to bed, then maybe I'll have a lighter dinner. If I'm going to go to aerobics class after dinner, then of course I'm going to fuel my body to get me through that class to the best of my ability.

• •

MAKE IT FUN!

Think of ways to make exercise fun for you. You can get certain results at the gym, but if the thought of going fills you with dread, then go outside and take a walk instead. Or grab your kids or your friends or the dog and go to the park. Throw a ball around or, even better, get a weighted ball. I bought a weighted hula hoop, which I love. Find ways to be active that you enjoy.

ships is part of the process of getting healthy, and I needed to work on my relationships now that I had some safe boundaries. So I started going out socially again, but with a big difference: I didn't go out every weekend, and I didn't drink alcohol. I just drank water—but boy, did I dance! I used to think I needed a few drinks to even consider getting out on the floor. I used to always say, "Oh, I'm not a very good dancer," or, "I dance better when I drink." But I never knew how much fun it could be just to dance. And I actually had great conversations with my friends that I could remember the next day! Not drinking made a huge difference in my overall health.

In general, I was just spending more time with the people I love, and I was having good, real conversations. I spent time with my niece Avery. I went hiking with my family. I made friends in my stepmom's biking group. I made friends at the gym who went biking and swimming with me. I just participated in a lot of different kinds of social environments. And I was wearing a bathing suit again! It felt so good to be back in the water.

A PHONE CALL

I had been home about 7 weeks and was still focused on becoming the at-home winner of *The Biggest Loser*. I used to fuss at Mom in the gym when she wasn't concentrating on her workouts. "Mom, get on the machine!" I'd scold her. "Why should I?" she'd respond. "You're going to win the $100,000 at-home prize, and I'm going to collect half of it."

One day Mom and I were in the locker room at the gym, and I got a phone call from the show's producers. They said they were calling all the eliminated contestants to give us another shot at being back on the ranch. When I hung up the phone, I looked at my mom.

"Oh my God. I'm going to be the first female Biggest Loser. I really am," I said. "I'm really going to do this."

"I know," she said.

An energy just rushed through my body. I felt it; I really did.

At the ranch, I had said I was going to win the title, but I can't say I really believed it and owned it until week 4—then I was eliminated. Once I got back home and refocused after that first night of "the old Ali," I began to own the goal to my very core. *I may not be able to compete for the title,* I thought, *but I'm going to show up with the highest weight loss percentage.* The result was that I worked out as if I had a shot at being the Biggest Loser one way or another. I wanted to do the impossible. Everyone said a woman couldn't do it, and I used that disbelief as fuel. I thrived on it. Don't tell me a woman can't do it. And now it looked like I had a shot at the actual title once again.

I didn't know what it would take to win a place back on the show. They didn't tell us what sort of challenge or test we would have to pass. Since I hadn't been the strongest competitor in the challenges, I hired a coach to do running drills with me. I believed in finding resources to help me build strength in my weak areas, and running was definitely one of my weaker areas. I worked on sprints and endurance. I kept saying to myself over and over, *I'm going to do this. I'm going to do it, or I'm going to die trying to get back on that ranch.*

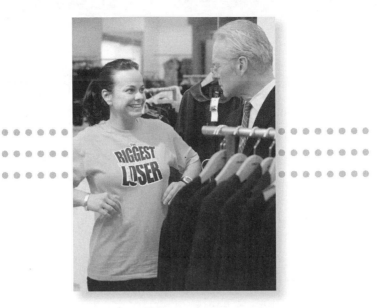

SIX

"Now I Believe!"

"You're going to do it, aren't you?"
—*Biggest Loser* crew member to Ali Vincent

W hen Mom and I got back to L.A. and saw the other eliminated contestants, we couldn't believe how amazing everyone looked. I remember seeing Amanda Harmer and thinking, "Wow—she's so skinny!" And when Mark Kruger got off the elevator, I didn't even recognize him. I was happy for everyone, but I have to admit, part of me was thinking, "Did I do enough?" I wasn't sure I had lost enough weight to win a place back at the ranch. And some people were still playing the game, being very secretive about how much weight they had lost.

Mom was out of her mind excited to be back at the ranch, to show me off. It felt good that she was so proud of me, but it also intensified the pressure I was feeling already with everyone checking me out. I didn't want the glare on me quite so intensely; I wanted to tell her to quit tooting my horn so much!

At dinner that night, we all wondered how the show's producers would choose who got to stay, what the criteria would be. Some of us even thought maybe they'd keep the person who had lost the least amount of weight, because that person would need time on the ranch the most. We had no idea what was coming.

NERVOUS AND SCARED

Back at the ranch, the group of us who had just returned to campus were kept behind a screen as the six remaining contestants filed into the weigh-in room. The guys still in the competition were Dan Evans, Roger Shultz, and Jay Kruger, and the remaining women were Maggie King, Brittany Aberle, and Kelly Fields. After we were revealed to those six, we found out that we would all weigh in, and the man and woman from our group with the highest percentages of weight loss would get to come back to the ranch. The order of the weigh-in was the same as the order in which we'd been eliminated. We had to wear our sports bras and bike shorts again, while the other contestants were covered up in their *Biggest Loser* tank tops. So here I was, back to feeling vulnerable. I wore a T-shirt over my sports bra, and I was placed in the back row. I remember seeing the ranch contestants craning their necks, trying to catch a glimpse of what I looked like. I was nervous and scared. It seemed like there was all this judgment in the air, a different energy from when I'd left 7 weeks ago—and there was definitely more game play.

When I took off my shirt to walk up to the scale, I could hear people whispering.

I stepped on the scale. I felt like I was in a fog, and then I heard my mom cry out "Yay!" as the scale registered a 67-pound weight loss, putting me in first place for the women. But it wasn't until the last woman, Jackie Evans, weighed in that I knew for sure that I had won myself a place back on the ranch. I think I felt every possible emotion at that moment.

As I stood with the group of contestants who would be staying at the ranch, I had never been more scared in my life. I looked at my mom, who was with the other eliminated contestants. I had never been on *The Biggest Loser* campus without her—and now I wanted her back! Even though I watched her walk out of the gym with everyone else, it didn't really sink in that she was gone until I was back in my room, lying alone on my bed and looking across at her empty bed. I was by myself. But I realized this: I had to finish this journey on my own. There were no excuses anymore. I didn't have Mom to worry about or our issues to distract me.

"Okay, Ali," I said to myself. "Here's the opportunity to be the woman you know is inside of you."

Later, everyone was asking me all kinds of questions about what I had been doing at home—how I had been eating, whether I'd been working out a lot. I answered honestly but wasn't sure about the intention behind their questions. These were the people who had sent me home. They were being nice, but they were also trying to figure me out. They were playing the game.

I was glad to be back. I tried to convey to everyone the lessons I'd learned from being eliminated—that we were all going home eventually and our journeys were so much bigger than day-to-day ranch politics and alliances. Everyone seemed to be so steeped in the game play that they weren't seeing the big picture. I think that's why Mark Kruger and I bonded in those last few weeks. We had both gone home, even though he only spent a week there. When he saw his family, he realized that they were the real reason he was doing this. It wasn't about the other contestants.

• •

WE ALL GO HOME EVENTUALLY

Bob and Jillian are at the ranch to help everyone succeed—and that success is not necessarily winning. Their most important job isn't helping someone win, but making sure each contestant figures out what has stopped them in the past and is able to find a way to live differently in the future.

• •

Mom and I were supposed to appear on the *Today* show together the week after I got back to the ranch. She had to go without me and because it was a secret that I was back in the competition, she just told the producers I was "otherwise engaged." I thought that was hilarious. I had never even been to New York City, but I couldn't make it to the *Today* show because of a prior engagement? While she was in New York, she bought me a little bell with apples on it and sent it to me at the ranch with a tag attached that said, "Believe It, Be It."

STAYING PINK

I had missed the whole part of the game when the contestants were divided up into two teams—blue and black—so it never occurred to me to choose to be black or blue once I was back. I was pink. And I was staying pink. It was just me. And we were competing as individuals again. I cared about everyone and just wanted to stay as neutral as possible.

I knew that Kelly, Brittany, and Maggie were upset that I was back, that any woman was back. But I also knew that I was there for a reason, even if it was just to spend some more time with the people on the ranch, particularly with the team I was training with, Jillian's team. These women were amazing, beautiful women, full of strength. But they were just so scared; they were scared to go home. That's how I felt the first time I was on the ranch—I was always worried about falling below the yellow line. But being away from the ranch gave me perspective and, I think, an advantage. When I got back, I didn't obsess about falling below the yellow line like I used to. I just focused on what I could control and did my best.

But Jillian saw things a little differently—and that first week back was definitely a test of wills between us. I understood that she was upset with me for continuing to wear my pink shirt and not joining her black team. She was trying to point out to me that while I may have been successful at home, being on the ranch is a whole different thing. People come to the ranch to build relationships, create amazing bonds with one another—and she seemed to think I was trying to separate myself from that. But from my perspective, while I was so grateful to be working out with incredible trainers and spending time with such wonderful people, at the end of the day I live my own life. And I had to figure that out. Staying in pink was part of that.

• •

SPEAK OUT

One night on the ranch I was in the gym and I felt like Jillian had forgotten about me as she focused on training some of the other contestants. In the past, I would not have said anything. I would have let the resentment build and collected evidence that here was yet another example of how I was unworthy. Instead, I reminded her that she hadn't trained me that evening. She apologized and then gave me an hour of one-on-one training. That night was probably one of my biggest breakthroughs on the ranch.

• •

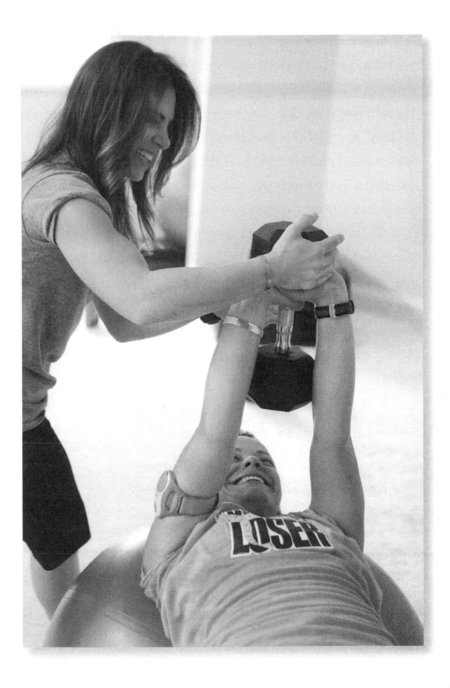

The first few workouts were tough, but I got through them. I needed to prove to myself that I wasn't going to die under Jillian's training, and she actually gave me some praise after one of our first workouts together. I remember her saying, "God, I'm just proud of you. I want to punch you out, I'm so proud." I think she was excited to have me back, and I think she knew that when I came back to the ranch and picked her to train with, she had her first female *Biggest Loser* winner!

It was an emotional time for the other women on the ranch. Some of them seemed to stop keeping close tabs on everything they ate—like forgetting to account for snacks—and those are the kinds of small things that can definitely catch up with you. You have to track every single thing you eat if you want to keep posting big numbers on the scale each week. They were feeling over-

• •

Visualize It

Those last few weeks on the ranch, I used to ask Jillian what she was going to wear on the *Today* show after I won *The Biggest Loser*. "Oh, Ali," she'd say. "You need to focus on your cycling!" And I told her I needed to focus on what we'd be wearing after I won so that I *could* cycle! If I thought about how hard she was going to make me spin, my body would cramp up. But if I thought about what I'd wear in my moment of glory, I'd spin my heart out! If you can focus on what you're going to create out of all your hard work, you can push through tough moments.

• •

• •

LET YOUR MIND CATCH UP

When you lose a lot of weight, it sometimes takes time for your mind to catch up with the changes that are taking place in the rest of your body. That happened to me in my makeover episode. I remember watching Heba Salama on Season 6 react to the size of dress that designer Christian Siriano (of *Project Runway* fame) had picked out for her. She immediately said, "I'll try it, but it's not going to fit." And did it ever fit! I remember that anxiety. Give yourself the time to get used to your new body, and don't be afraid to try new things. That's part of the fun!

• •

whelmed by the pressure of weighing in against the men, afraid the odds were stacked against them—and then I appeared and changed the game even more for them.

When I weighed in at the end of that first week back, I won. I beat all the guys. And in fact, I won every other weigh-in after I got back, except for one.

I just decided to go for it. That's what you have to do with any goal or difficult journey. I did everything that was asked of me and then some. I tracked the calories I ate in my food journal and in and out on my Bodybugg. I put in the workout time. I never stopped. When I wasn't working out, I walked. Unless I was sleeping, I never sat still. I just stayed busy doing different things. I knew that's what had worked for me at home, and I thought, *I'm just going to keep doing that.* I had become active again in all aspects of my life. I no longer wanted to simply sit around or veg out in front of the TV. Honestly, I still don't. I don't even go to see movies much anymore, because I can always get on the treadmill and pop in a DVD or watch a TV show while I cycle. I just like to stay moving.

I FEEL PRETTY

During my second week back at the ranch, we filmed the makeover episode. I had only recently started to realize how much my body had changed. I had noticed the internal changes all along—I was stronger and could make it through a day with more energy—but for a long time I felt like I just looked like a smaller version of the big me. But now I was starting to look longer and leaner. I could see in the mirror that my face had started to change shape. I was feeling good about myself—and sexy! I was proud of myself again. And the great thing about the makeover show is that it really allows you to appreciate how far you've come—your mind gets a chance to catch up with all the changes in your body.

We met up with *Project Runway* host Tim Gunn at Macy's in Los Angeles. We had to get up at 3:00 in the morning to be at Macy's and ready to tape by 5:00 a.m.! They needed to shoot the episode when the store was empty. Of course, I took my sleep mask and pillow with me and napped during the van ride.

Tim Gunn was so gracious and friendly. After we met him, we walked around the store and looked at clothes we might like.

Then he joined us, gave us feedback about what he thought suited us, and helped us pick out some outfits. I knew I had lost weight, but I was still scared to try on the smaller sizes, because I didn't want to feel bad if they didn't fit! But I ended up going down *four dress sizes* before I found something that fit. I had no idea that I was so much smaller. Tim kept saying, "I think you're this size," and I would say, "No, I think I'm a bigger size."

I had an image in my mind of the kind of dress I wanted to wear—a sort of modern twist on a classic, Audrey Hepburn look. I wanted to be sexy but not over the top. So Tim picked out an empire-waist dress for me, cream with black lace and spaghetti straps. I almost swooned. I hadn't gone sleeveless for years! Even on the days at the ranch when the cameras weren't rolling and the other girls would wear tank tops, I never did. It was one of my dreams, to lose enough weight to proudly bare my arms, and here I was at that moment. When I saw the dress on the mannequin, I thought it was too beautiful for me to put on. I just looked at it, thinking it was the sort of thing I'd always wanted to wear but never felt I could. I started crying.

We were pampered the entire day. We had our hair and makeup done, and I decided to have all my hair cut off! Here I was, the hairstylist letting go of all my hair. It was very symbolic for me. I had kept my hair long because I didn't feel I could pull off the short, funky cuts that I always liked. I got a wonderful bob with bangs and felt terrific.

After our hair and makeup was complete, we found out that

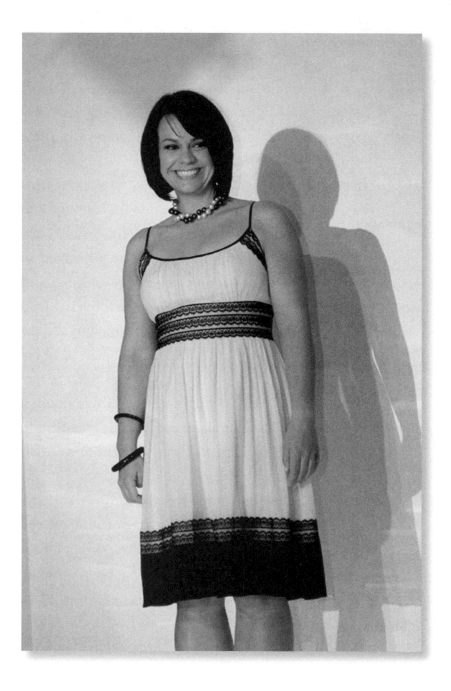

we were going to be part of a fashion show, so we had to practice walking up and down a runway. A room had been set up with tables and chairs and a runway. I went up and down the runway concentrating on my moves, practicing a sassy walk and putting my hand on my hip, and when I looked up, there at the end of the runway stood my sister Amber! I burst into tears and ran toward her. We hugged, and she said, "I have my sister back." Then I stood back so that she could see me, and I pointed to my collarbone. "Look, I have a collarbone!" I said. The other contestants were reunited with their family members as well, and then we all sat down together to celebrate the special day with sparkling apple cider. It had been so long since I had been around my sister and had felt good about myself. I was strong, fit, and alive. For years, I had been happy for Amber but also jealous. I didn't want to be jealous of her anymore. I just wanted to love her.

By my third week back on campus, I had lost a total of 85 pounds, the most any woman had lost to date at that point in *Biggest Loser* history. I weighed 149 pounds. It felt amazing. I was doing things that worked for me. I wasn't playing the game, I was just working hard and controlling the things I could control. Even the crew members started to believe I could do it. Usually they didn't speak to us, but after one particularly grueling challenge in which the guys kind of ganged up on Kelly and me, one of the crew members turned to me and said,

"Damn, girl, you're going to do it, aren't you? Now *I* believe!"

EXCESS SKIN

I've gotten a lot of e-mails from women asking about having extra skin after losing all that weight. Young women have told me they want to quit losing weight because they're starting to see their skin sag. I think that's a shame, especially since they were getting healthy.

Some *Biggest Loser* contestants do choose to have skin removal surgery after they've lost the weight. But the scars that come with it are substantial. I guess if you're going to have a scar as a reminder of your weight loss battle, that's a way to look at it—as a battle wound. If I ever have babies, maybe I'll have a tummy tuck. But I just don't focus on excess skin right now. I have a beautiful body, I'm healthy, and I'm strong.

I remember during the final weeks of being on the ranch, I was lying on my bed, looking at my legs. I had started to pay more attention to my body. I have big calves, and I was thinking—maybe for a split second—"I could get calf reduction surgery." And then I thought, "These are my calves, and they're fine. And I'm not going to worry what someone else thinks about them." I kind of think that's what you have to do with the focus on excess skin, or anything else that bothers you about your body. What's really important is your health.

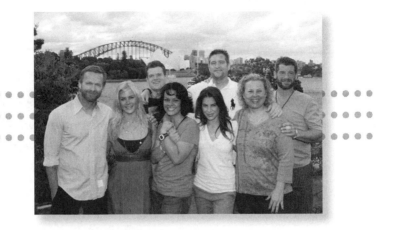

SEVEN

Where Rainbows Begin

I was having an out-of-body experience.

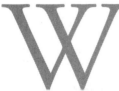e were in the elimination room at the end of my fourth week back on the campus, week 14 in TV time. Dan had just been eliminated, so it was down to the final five: Roger, Jay, Mark, Kelly, and me. Ali Sweeney asked us to stay in the elimination room after Dan left, which was unusual. We waited anxiously, wondering what kind of twist she was about to announce. Then she told us something we never would have

• •

WHO INSPIRES YOU?

One way to stay motivated is to think about who inspires you. My mom inspires me. She went to that ranch with me and endured lots of hard, tough changes. Trainers inspire me—seeing them work out with people and push them to their limits. Watching athletes compete in competitions like the Ironman or the Olympics inspires me. Who inspires you?

• •

guessed: We were leaving for Australia where we would compete in a triathlon!

I was so excited. I'd heard stories my whole life about my grandmother growing up in New Zealand, and now I was going to see that part of the world for the first time. My grandma was 84, and she hadn't been home since she was 26. I felt lucky to have the opportunity to visit a place so far away. I couldn't wait to get there. I was ready to start my new life.

THIS WAS A NIGHT

Bob and Jillian met us in Sydney and decided to take us out for a night on the town before all of the hard work began. The only problem was, I didn't have a thing to wear! I had been living in a pair of size 12 jeans that I'd borrowed from my sister's friend while I was home after my week 4 elimination. Holly had put out an SOS for clothes—anything from a 4 to 14—when I was home, because as I lost weight, I was losing my wardrobe. When her friend gave me those jeans, I could barely zip them. And now in Australia, just a few weeks later, they were practically falling off my body! I had cinched them around my waist with a belt so they wouldn't just slide off my hips. Faced with a big night out, I was definitely feeling frumpy.

We had half an hour to run into a store and get something to wear for our night out. It was the first time in my adult life that I was able to just grab something off a rack that I wanted to wear—and it fit! I got the cutest black silky shirt with ruffles and a pair of skinny jeans. I was in and out of the store in 15 minutes with an outfit. It was an amazing feeling to be able to find something so quickly that looked good on me—something I wanted to wear. Roger told me later I looked smoking hot. Even Bob was like, "Damn!" I felt like the hottest thing ever!

Here I was in flipping Sydney, Australia. I had just popped into a boutique and bought a new outfit, and now we were going out to dinner at one of the nicest restaurants in Sydney. It was

• •

SALAD SCENARIO

A common mistake people make when eating out is assuming that the best choice is always a salad. But restaurant salads can be loaded with fattening dressing and cheese. A better choice, I think, is grilled chicken or fish with lots of steamed veggies.

• •

• •

WHAT ABOUT DRINKING?

Is drinking alcohol bad? No, not in moderation. But if you're trying to lose weight, be careful. One drink often leads to two or three, and when your inhibitions are lowered, it's easy to overeat.

• •

crazy expensive, a place I would never go under normal circumstances. But Bob and Jillian were treating! We went out dancing afterward, and it felt like a night of celebration. We had a triathlon and a weigh-in coming up, but that night, we were celebrating the success we had already achieved.

Sydney is such a beautiful city. There are these fabulous markets everywhere that sell every kind of fresh fruit and vegetable imaginable, and the people there are so active—it seemed like everyone was outdoors enjoying the amazing weather. We burned a lot of our calories just sightseeing and walking. We still worked out and ran, but we did a lot of activities outside.

A CHALLENGE FOR ATHLETES

Our challenge for the week was to compete in a triathlon (though I called it a quadrathlon, because it was broken up into four parts). We started on top of Sydney Harbor Bridge. When we looked out over the bridge, we could see the opera house and the harbor, just like you see on TV. At first we thought our challenge was just going to be climbing up the bridge. Then Alison Sweeney told us that first we would have to swim across Sydney Harbor, then we would bike through a park, run to an office building, and finally climb 40 flights of stairs to the top and cross the finish line. I loved swimming and biking, and I was learning to love running. So I felt ready for the challenge.

The only tricky part for me about the swimming: It was in open water. I'm a pool swimmer—I like to be able to see the drain. In a pool, your body is parallel to the surface, and you're really gliding through the water, making small rotations to get your breath as you constantly stroke. In open water, you have to kind of sit up to breathe, because there's a current and waves, so there's always water splashing in your face. You have to get above the water and bob up to breathe, so you don't choke.

I started out that race swimming freestyle. But I couldn't see clearly in the murky water, and I started to panic. I felt like I was suffocating. I began to think, *I can't do this.* I had to talk myself through the fear and reassure myself that I'd be okay. *Just calm down,* I thought. *You're a strong, capable woman.* Then it occurred to me to flip over onto my back and try swimming the backstroke. Once I did that, I was able to relax. I quit hyperventilating, and I started to enjoy looking up at the sky. It was beautiful. And I made it to the end of the swim that way, on my back.

When I got out of the water, I was in the lead by about a minute and 45 seconds. The cycling part was next. But we couldn't just hop on our bikes. We had to run up stairs to find our bikes, and that's when Mark caught up with me. But I was okay with it. I had been running with Mark and was getting better at it, but I knew it wasn't my strong point. Once we were on our bikes, he passed me. I was still in second place, but there's something about being ahead—when you have the lead, it seems like it's easier to keep it. When you're lagging behind, it becomes tough to overtake the person ahead of you. But I just kept pushing, I never gave up. Next we raced through the botanical garden, and I started gaining on Mark. I remember running past an older man in the park who yelled out to me, "Stop losing weight! You look great!" It was nice to have a stranger cheering me on.

Finally, we got to the office building. I just put my head down and was determined to do it. It was very humid—it was summer in Australia—and as an Arizona girl, I'm used to heat but not humidity. I was sweaty and hot and parched. But I was going up those stairs, and I was giving it everything I had. When I was on about the fourth or fifth floor, I looked up and thought, "Oh my God, I'm going to die. How am I going to do this?" I was utterly exhausted. When I was finally nearing the top of the staircase, I saw Mark just standing there. He was waiting for me.

"What are you doing?" I asked him.

He grinned and said, "I need help getting to the top."

"Shut up," I said. "No, you don't."

"I can't cross the finish line," he said.

"Well, then," I said, "get on my back, damn it."

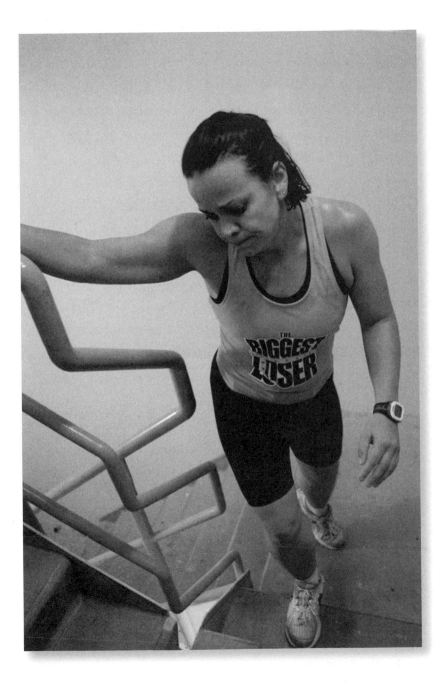

I was so exhausted that I was shaking, but I was moved that he had waited for me. We crossed the finish line together, me carrying him on my back. At that point, we had both won. Neither of us needed to cross first. It really didn't matter. What mattered was our experience on this journey, our memories, our moments—enjoying every second and celebrating how far we'd come.

GOD HIMSELF

Because we won together, Mark and I got to share the reward for the triathlon challenge, which was a seaplane ride to a beautiful cliff-top restaurant. The view was amazing—it looked as if God himself had designed each bit of it, saying, "Oh, I think a cloud should go here and some water would be good there. . . . Done, done, done." I can't describe that part of the world. I'd never seen such green. I wasn't used to it, the trees, the colors. It was like a painting.

When we landed, Mark and I had breakfast and just took it all in. Then we were each given 15 minutes to call our families from a cell phone. I immediately called my grandma's number. My mom picked up. She kept trying to talk to me about what was going on in the competition, but the funny thing was, I didn't care. I just told her, "Mom, I don't want to talk about it." At that moment, my life was about celebration. Sure, it was about pushing myself to my limits, but it was also about celebrating and enjoying and sensing . . . acknowledging the different smells and colors.

• •

CONSISTENT EFFORT

As a contestant, I was never the one to do anything particularly out of the ordinary, but I was the one who was consistent and steady. Consistency is key when you're trying to make big changes in your life.

• •

Then I talked to Grandma. I told her how beautiful her part of the world was, and she told me how proud she was of me and that she loved me—but not to come home before the finals! She said that my mom was okay and not to worry about her. She said I should just do what I needed to do.

I felt like I was having an out-of-body experience. It was just so beautiful. And that was when I saw a rainbow coming out of the water. I watched a rainbow begin to form. It was one of those moments in life you never forget; it was so special. I felt strong, capable, beautiful, generous, loving, and loved. I felt amazing.

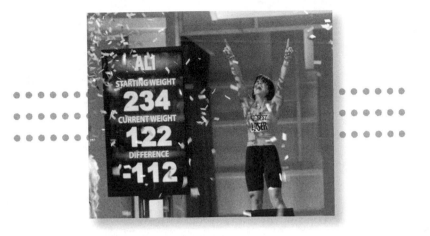

EIGHT

This Is My Night, and I'm Going to Own It like No Other

Of course it's hard, because it wouldn't feel this good if it weren't.

I'm a great believer in the power of collecting evidence for success. When I was overweight and felt stuck, I'd collect evidence that supported my excuses for why everything wasn't how I wanted it to be. I'd say, "Oh, I just don't fit in," or, "I'm not being judged fairly." I was always looking to the negative to explain away my unhappiness. But as I lost the weight, I got into the habit of collecting positive evidence, of looking for all the reasons why I *could* succeed.

When I was living with Holly back in Arizona after Mom and I had been eliminated, Holly was about 8 months pregnant. She and I were close, but we'd never been as close as we became during that time. When she had her first baby—my niece Avery—I'd been at the hospital to support Holly, but not actually with her in the delivery room. Before I found out I was going back to *The Biggest Loser* ranch, Holly had asked me if I would be with her when she had her daughter Macy. It was an amazing and touching request that I was thrilled to accept, but then, when I found out I was going back to the ranch, I realized I would be away for her delivery. I told her how sorry I was that I was going to miss the birth of my second niece. But Holly said, "You know what, Ali? I'm going to have plenty of babies, so don't think about that. You go and do this."

After we completed the triathalon in Australia, we were all anxious about the upcoming weigh-in. We didn't know what effect the travel would have on our bodies. On the day of the weigh-in—February 19—I got the news that Macy had been born! She was healthy and beautiful, and Holly's delivery had been quick and problem free. And it turned out that it was not only my new niece's birthday—but it also happened to be Jillian's birthday. When I saw Jillian right before the weigh-in, she was stressed out, nervous about how I was going to do. I just looked at her and said, "Jill, we're going to be okay. Don't worry. My sister just had a baby on your birthday." It was like an omen to me. I didn't have to worry. I was collecting evidence for my success. Everything was going to be okay.

None of us did great at that weigh-in—most people lost only a pound or two. I was the winner, with a 3-pound weight loss. It was a tough situation for brothers Mark and Jay, who fell below the yellow line. Big brother Mark had gone home earlier in the competition, giving up hs spot at the ranch so that his brother could stay. This time Jay stepped up to the plate and went home, giving Mark a second chance.

We had only 1 more week to go on the ranch before our last weigh-in. Then the final three would go home for several weeks before the live finale. When we got back to the ranch from our trip, Alison Sweeney told us that we'd be working out by ourselves that week, without the help of our trainers.

"You think you can do it again, Ali?" she said. "Can you pull it off? You have one more weigh-in . . . "

"No, Alison, I have two more weigh-ins," I told her. "The one coming up and then the finale. And yes, I plan on winning both."

Mark, Kelly, Roger, and I were the final four. And Roger, a big guy and former football player, said he planned on losing 15 pounds that week to set a *Biggest Loser* weight loss record. That's a big number to pull the last, and 15th, week on campus. I was worried. I had been envisioning the finale, standing on that scale as the first female Biggest Loser, confetti falling down on me. The person who leaves the ranch with the highest percentage of weight loss gets to pick the order in which the finalists weigh in at the live finale. I knew that I wanted to step on the scale last, after everyone else, and have the confetti rain down on me. That's the way I had pictured it in my mind. I needed to win that last weigh-in to make it happen.

So I did the math. If Roger was going to lose 15 pounds, I needed to lose 9 pounds. I knew Roger would lose that amount and no more—he always did exactly what he said he was going to do. Mark and I went for a walk, weighed our chances, and tried to figure out the numbers. He didn't think he had enough weight left to lose to beat Roger, and he didn't think I could beat him, either.

THE LAST CHALLENGE

The last challenge was a relay race on the beach, with a twist: We had to wear a fat suit that was equal in weight to all the pounds we'd lost so far. For me, that meant putting 88 pounds back on my body. We had to run down the beach to a set of flags, pick up the one with our name on it, and then jog up to the top of a nearby mountain.

I was upset about putting on the fat suit. I just thought it was humiliating. I understood the intention behind the challenge, that it was a way for us to physically feel how much lighter we had

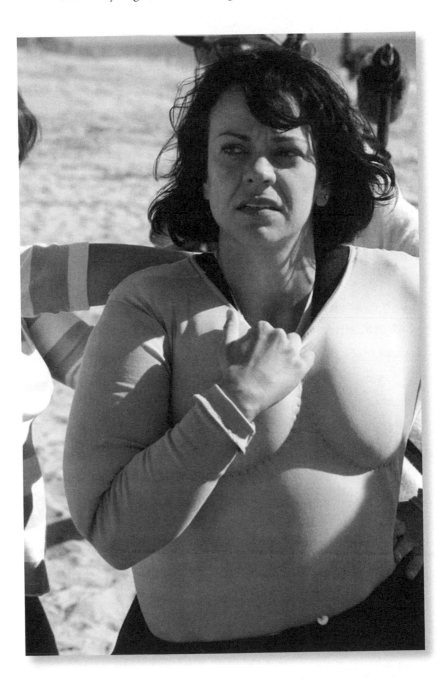

become and to appreciate how different our bodies were now, but I *never* wanted to feel what it was like to carry around all that weight again. I struggled when I put on my suit—the weighted vests were heavy against my chest. I felt like I couldn't breathe. And I couldn't believe this was the weight I used to carry around. It affected me physically and mentally. We were on a public beach, so as I literally waddled across the sand, people were watching. I hated it. This just wasn't me anymore.

As I made my way down the beach, shedding the weights, I relished feeling so much lighter. The energy came back into my body, like a rush of adrenaline. I remember running up the mountain for the last part of the challenge and holding my pink flag with "Ali" written across it. I felt triumphant! Like a superhero— look at me!

Overall, every challenge we competed in was worthwhile. As we got stronger and made it further along in the competition, our focus was less on winning the challenges and more on experiencing them and appreciating how far we'd come. They were hard. The whole process was hard. But you know what? It wouldn't have felt as good if it hadn't been.

THE FINAL RANCH WEIGH-IN

Before the final weigh-in on the ranch, we all assumed that only three of us would be going to the finale. That's how it had always worked on previous seasons of the show. Two women, two men, vying for three slots. Roger, with his vow to lose 15 pounds, weighed in first. And he'd done it. He'd lost 15 pounds, for a weight loss percentage of 6.41 percent.

Then Mark got on the scale, and he had lost an incredible 12 pounds. Starting the weigh-in at 182 pounds compared with Roger's 234, now *he* was in first place, with an astonishing weight loss percentage of 6.63 percent. Would my plan succeed? Had I made the numbers work? I was next. Heart pounding, I stepped up on the scale. I was starting at 146 pounds. I racked up an 11-pound loss, for a weight loss percentage of 7.53 percent! I was in first place! I could not stop smiling as I came down from the scale. I had lost a total of 99 pounds over the entire season, beating my own record for the most pounds lost by a woman on campus.

Last to weigh in was Kelly, who was terrified of what the scale would show. Starting at 191 pounds, she had dropped 13 pounds, for a weight loss percentage of 6.81 percent, putting her in second place. The women had swept the men! Kelly and I were jumping up and down and hugging Jillian. *We,* the women, were going to the finale, and *we* would decide who would be the third finalist between Mark and Roger, since they'd both fallen below the yellow line. That's the way it had worked in previous seasons. Right? Right?

No.

In one of those twists that only a reality TV show or just plain reality can deliver, Ali Sweeney told us that America would choose the third finalist to go to the finale. It was not up to the contestants who'd won the last weigh-in.

I was stunned. We all were. Jillian flipped out. Bob just stood there. We were all expecting that the rules would be the same as they were in previous seasons—none of us saw this coming. But I understood that it was all part of the game, a game I'd chosen to be a part of. So I calmed myself down and thought, "Okay, here we go. It's just another bump in the road. I'll deal with it." The threat was that Roger still had a lot of weight left to lose.

The time had come for us to go home for about 5 weeks before we came back to California for the live finale. Leaving *The Biggest Loser* campus was bittersweet. I knew I was ending one part of my journey and embarking on another. I was closing a chapter in my life, but I was looking forward to the next chapters, to setting new goals, to building on what I had learned. The ranch is where I learned to dream again. It's where I learned how to celebrate me and how to push myself further than I thought I could ever go. I knew that I would draw strength from the experiences I'd had there for the rest of my life, and that I'd finally be able to create the kind of future I wanted, now that I had the tools and the motivation to do so.

There had been many moments in my past that I hadn't really been present for. I was checked out. But during my entire time on *The Biggest Loser* ranch, I made such an effort to be present, to be open and vulnerable. To take everything in and breathe it in. When I walked around the ranch, I found myself noticing everything around me—the trees and the squirrels and the rocks underneath my feet. I felt like I was part of the world again.

I remembered the words of that producer, back in the hotel where the contestants for my season had been chosen. He told us that from that point on, we'd think of our lives in terms of "before" and "after" *The Biggest Loser*. He was right.

COMING HOME AGAIN

As I was driven from the airport to my dad's house in Chandler, Arizona, I was excited to see my family, but I was also nervous and scared. I'd had a lot of "me" time on the ranch. And while I'd been back there for only 6 weeks, those weeks had been priceless to me. I wasn't sure how much my family would notice the physical changes. But I wanted them to recognize how much I had changed on the inside. Those last few weeks at the ranch and in Australia had been hugely spiritual for me. Would the people who'd known me my whole life—who knew the old me—be open

• •

FOOD AS A FIX

The next time you find yourself mindlessly standing in front of the refrigerator or the cupboard or your snack drawer, ask yourself if you're really hungry. When was the last time you ate? Maybe just drink a glass of water first. You might be mistaking thirst for hunger. Then think about what may have triggered an urge to snack. Did you just get in a fight with your mom? Did you just have a confrontation with a colleague? Figure out what you're trying to fix and deal with it.

• •

and responsive to the new me? Or would they try to pull me back into the version of me they were comfortable with?

I was also harboring my own doubts about being able to go all the way. As much as I felt in my heart that I was going to win, I also knew that many times in my life I'd gone 99.9 percent of the distance toward achieving a goal, only to pull back at the very end. Was I going to be able to do this? To finish? Or would the pressure be too much for me?

When we pulled up to the house, I saw a long pink carpet leading up to the front door. As I entered the backyard, I was overwhelmed by how many people had come to share and celebrate this moment with me. Everyone I knew was there, cheering and tossing rose petals. Amber was there, which completely surprised me because she had just visited me in L.A., and since she was a mom with two young kids at home, I knew it wasn't easy for her to travel. Both my grandmothers were there, too, and of course, my parents. All these people had gotten together and planned this for me—I had never experienced anything like it. I didn't have a graduation party; I'd never had a wedding. I'd never had any kind of a celebration where this many people came out to support me. And there I was with all these people who love me—family, friends, extended family, extended friends. Even my dad's friends were there, telling me how much I had inspired them. And everything was pink! Everyone wore pink shirts, gave me pink flowers—there was even pink punch to drink! My brothers collected

99 pounds of fat from butchers and Dumpsters and put it in a pink wheelbarrow. Everyone just made such a big effort. It was pure celebration.

So that was the fun night. Starting the next day, I really began to feel the pressure. I didn't want to disappoint all these people who were so proud of me. The feelings of self-doubt started to creep in. I was letting the pressure overwhelm me. I became worried that I was going to sabotage myself. And while I didn't crash and burn, I did start to find myself doing things I shouldn't, like standing in front of the freezer at night, dipping into the frozen yogurt for another spoonful when I wasn't hungry.

Everywhere I went in my hometown, people followed me. In the grocery store, I could feel them watching what I put in my basket. At the gym, people approached me to ask questions when I was working out. I was happy to share my experience with everyone and encourage them, but I also needed to focus.

I had a little bit of an advantage over the other contestants: I had already been through this. I'd set up a program the first time I was home that had worked for me, so I just went right back to what I'd done before. I moved in with Holly and Andy again. I childproofed my life (from myself, not my nieces!) to keep temptations at bay and avoided tempting situations. I lived on a calorie budget and a schedule. I made lots of lists. My life had structure. As Jillian says, if you fail to plan, you plan to fail.

I had my trainers and my gym and my classes. I made a conscious decision to compete like I had never competed before. This was my Olympic gold medal, my Tour de France. I chose to compete like an athlete. I would give it everything I had.

I was determined to follow through and accomplish my goal. So I had to figure out why I was dipping into the frozen yogurt at night and why I seemed to be tempted to give up at the finish line. And here is what I realized: Having a finish line in front of me represented the end of something. I was so close to the finale, the end, and I didn't know what would come next. So I had to start thinking about that: What would I do next? In the past, I'd gone on diets, but once I got to a certain place, I would quit. I didn't plan for the next steps. So I realized maybe I would have to plan for what came next. I was an athlete, and I knew that athletes train for specific goals and events. I needed goals. I needed something to train for, look forward to, and celebrate when it was over. Once I got that, it clicked. I was able to wrap my mind around finishing this part of my life, because it would just be the first of many challenges I would embrace.

Have you ever waited in line for a scary ride at a fair or an amusement park, and right as you're about to step up for your turn, you notice a little gate off to one side—the "chicken exit"? It's your last chance to pull out, even if you waited in line half the day and looked forward to the thrill. I didn't want to have any chicken exits in my life. I wanted to go to that finale, and if I didn't win, it wouldn't be because I was too afraid to get on the ride. If I didn't win, it just meant I didn't win.

When I was younger, I had taken the chicken exit many times. In swimming, I was naturally talented and I practiced, but I had those days when I cut practice or didn't do all the land drills I was supposed to do. That way, there would be a reason if I didn't win a competition—I could count on knowing I hadn't done everything I could. That was my excuse. But I didn't want an excuse anymore. I didn't want to operate my life like that. Chicken exits are self-sabotage. They give you a false explanation for why you don't have something you want. Up until this point in my life, I had never given anything all that I had to give. But I was going to now.

HEADING BACK FOR THE FINALE

I'd planned for my big finale moment for months, and in great detail. I knew how I wanted everything to look, from my hair to

. . . .

LOSING THE LAST 10 POUNDS

Jillian calls the last 10 pounds "vanity pounds." Back when I had more than 100 pounds to lose and I heard ladies talking about losing those last 10 pounds, I'd think, "That's just sand off the dunes." But when I got to my last 10 pounds before the finale, I understood. It's *hard* to lose them! And I found out how do it—you push yourself even harder. You do that by upping the ante. On the treadmill, for example, you step it up a notch. If you're at 5 miles per hour, go to 5.5. If you're at an incline setting of 6, nudge it up to 6.3. You have to push past your comfort zone to get to your goal weight.

. . . .

my makeup to my outfit, and I didn't leave anything to chance. I had my makeup done the day before the finale in a test run. This was my day! It was like my wedding day. The morning of the show, I had my makeup artist and hairstylist come to my hotel room early and get me ready.

The show's wardrobe department picks out really nice clothes for the contestants to choose from, but by now, you know me! I had my vision, and I wanted to wear something I absolutely loved for my big moment. I went shopping with some friends and told them what I was looking for—a dress, form-fitting but classy, with clean lines. Something that showed off my newly buff arms and my collarbone. As I described what I wanted, my friend Tina said she had the perfect dress at home and she'd be happy to lend it to me.

Now, Tina is my skinny friend. "I'm never going to fit into anything you own," I told her. But she insisted, so we went to her apartment. She showed me the dress, which was Italian, stretchy, and tiny. I went into the bathroom to try it on, not knowing how it was going to turn out, and . . . oh my God, that dress fit perfectly. I just couldn't believe it. I came out and looked at myself in her mirror and knew that I had found my dress. I wanted a belt to go with it, a touch of pink. My sister Holly had a great pink belt she'd worn while she was pregnant, so we just lopped off part of the belt and attached a fun pink feather.

I was also having a hard time finding the perfect shoes. I had seen a beautiful pair of pink Christian Louboutins with little ruffles in the back, but Oprah had just featured his shoes on her show, and the demand was so overwhelming that they were back-ordered. So I bought some black patent leather heels with peep toes, and my sister glued tiny pink Swarovski crystals all over the heels.

I even borrowed jewelry to complete my look. I hadn't been able to find anything I liked at the shops I went to in Phoenix. Then a friend offered to let me borrow her ring, which was a big pink topaz surrounded by little sapphires. It was beautiful. I called it the Ring of the First Female Biggest Loser. (I have one just like it today.) I went online to look at more jewelry from the boutique where my friend had gotten her ring and saw a pair of earrings and a necklace that were exactly what I had been looking for. But they were so expensive! So the next day—and this was literally a day before I was leaving for the finale—I called the jewelry store and explained my situation to a complete stranger.

"Hi, you don't know me, but my name's Ali Vincent, and I'm about to win a show called *The Biggest Loser,* and there's never been a female who's won it, so it's a pretty big deal. I'm going to be on live prime-time TV, and there's going to be a lot of press, and I'm going to be the one they're interviewing, because I'm going to win this thing. Is there any way you would loan me some jewelry to wear?"

The response? "Absolutely."

So there I had it! My finale ensemble was ready, complete with bedazzled shoes, borrowed dress, loaned jewelry, and a homemade belt! I felt like a Biggest Loser princess!

THE DAY OF THE FINALE

As we stood backstage watching the TV monitors, we waited for the results of America's vote between Mark and Roger as the third finalist to join the weigh-in with Kelly and me. Roger looked skinny. Alison Sweeney was wearing a microphone for TV, but it was hard for us to hear her unless you were standing close to the monitors. Bob and Jillian were standing with us, and Jillian leaned over to me and whispered, "You know if he's in, he wins," and I said, "I know." I didn't even look at her; I was just glued to the monitor, trying to hear what was going on.

And then Alison said, "America votes Roger!" and I literally dropped down into a ball, crouched down on my crystal-studded heels, bawling. Everybody thought the competition was Roger's to lose. It was such a weird experience; I felt like every part of my body was crying. Jillian came over and knelt down beside me and helped me stand back up. "You're going to be okay," she said. She hugged me. "You did it." I knew that she respected everything I'd been through. We are both women of passion and drive, who pursue our goals with steadfast determination. We had both given everything we had to this effort. It was our journey, and I was a changed woman. She was right; I had won, no matter what. We had pushed ourselves like nobody else. I knew I had given it everything.

So I just took a deep breath and calmed down, and that was it—there was nothing else to do. It was over. And it didn't matter, because I had done what I'd done for me. And for the first time in

● ●

ABOUT THE SCALE

My whole life, I got on the scale and I weighed in, and the numbers only ever went in one direction—up. On the ranch, we didn't have personal scales. So when I headed home for the first time, Bob counseled me not to get on the scale. He knew I could become obsessive about it and weigh myself several times a day. That doesn't help, since our bodies fluctuate throughout the day. If you want to weigh yourself, make regular dates with your scale, once a week at the same time of day and wearing the same type of clothing. But please, don't let the scale rule your life. When I quit living my life based on the number I saw on the scale, I took control of my body and my mind.

● ●

my life, I'd given 100 percent. I looked beautiful, and I felt beautiful. All my friends and family had come out to support me. Even Grandma was there. It was a big deal for her to come to the finale—she hadn't traveled in years, and it was exhausting for her. So I just decided that I was going to celebrate no matter what happened. I thought, "I may not be the first female Biggest Loser, but this is my night, and I'm going to own it like no other."

Before we weighed in, Kelly and I had been introduced to the audience in our dresses and high heels and makeup. We had to literally bust through life-size posters of ourselves at our original weights. The night before, we had rehearsed ripping through the paper. But as I stood behind that paper that night with a live audience waiting on the other side, I thought, "In 2.3 seconds, the whole world is going to judge me." I had my fists raised to punch through the paper, and then I saw the eyes on that poster. My eyes. They looked so sad and lost. I had a conversation with the old Ali. I told her, "You're okay. You are amazing and wonderful, and you will never feel the way you used to feel again. This change is for the rest of your life." I refused to punch my face, but I punched the hell out of that belly. *Pow!* I ripped right through and went out there on the stage and just owned it. It was so much fun! I don't remember ever having that much energy. It felt like every single childhood Christmas rolled into one.

MOMENT OF A LIFETIME

After we changed into our weigh-in clothes, I got to pick the order that Kelly, Roger, and I stepped on the scale, since I had left the ranch with the highest percentage of weight loss. I let Roger go first, then Kelly.

Roger had lost 164 pounds for a weight loss percentage of 45.18 percent. Kelly lost 109 pounds for a weight loss percentage of 40.22 percent. Roger's percentage was the number to beat.

Then it was my turn. I stepped on the scale. Alison told me I needed to have lost 105 pounds in order to win, so I knew what I was up against. It was crazy in that auditorium. Everyone was cheering and yelling. Up until that point, I had been thinking that Roger had won it. But 105 pounds? I thought, "I could still win this thing." But I still wouldn't believe it until I saw the num-

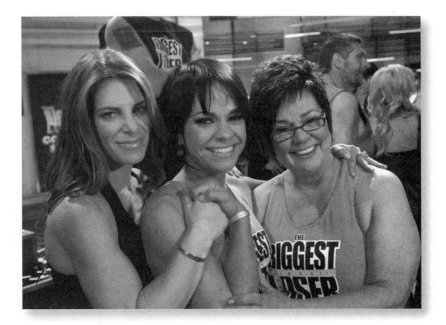

ber on the scale. When I looked down and saw that the scale showed 122 pounds, I was in such a flutter that I couldn't do the math. I had to turn around and look at the screen behind me to see that I had lost 112 pounds for the winning weight loss percentage of 47.86 percent! And then, just like I'd always pictured, the confetti started falling. I couldn't believe it. *I did it!* I raised my hands. I screamed. It was incredible.

It was the moment of a lifetime. I had never had that kind of moment, ever. The first person I hugged after getting down from the scale was my mom who was also up on the stage. But I had gotten an e-mail from Jillian earlier saying, "Just so we're clear and there are no mistakes, this is the way it breaks down. . . . I am the first person you hug." So she was the next person I grabbed, and soon all three of us were hugging, covered in confetti.

NO TIME TO CELEBRATE

As soon as the finale finished taping, we had to do an hour of press interviews, and then Jillian and I got on a red-eye flight to New York City so that we could be on the *Today* show the next morning. I practically had to be pulled out of that auditorium. I was trying to find my grandma and give her a kiss good-bye and say "I love you" to her and everyone else. My sisters helped me quickly gather all my things.

When we got to the airport to check in, Jillian realized I had a seat in coach while she was in first class. It didn't matter to me. I'd never flown first class in my life except for once, a few weeks earlier, when I had shot an ad for the milk campaign along with the other finalists—we'd all had our photos taken, and the winner of the show would have their ad featured in *USA Today* the day after the finale. Of course, I'd worn a pink dress for my shoot!

Jillian was ready for a fight to get me into first class. "You are my first female Biggest Loser, and you're *not* flying coach," she said. She threw down her credit card to pay for my first class ticket, and I was protesting all the way—I didn't want her to pay for me.

"Listen to me, and listen to me good," she said. "You need to get your rest, because tomorrow you're going to be on the *Today* show and you're going to be the first female Biggest Loser on it, and you're going to look good."

In the end, there were no more first class seats, so she gave me hers and got a business ticket for herself. The funny thing was, even in first class, I couldn't sleep. I was sitting next to an actor, and when the flight attendant announced on the PA system that the first female Biggest Loser was on the flight, he wouldn't stop talking to me!

When we landed at JFK, we ran through the airport to get to the car that was taking us to the *Today* show. I wanted to stop at a newsstand and see if my milk ad was in *USA Today*. I was dying to see it. "Oh, brother," Jillian said to me. So we stopped, and I grabbed a paper and started flipping through it, but I couldn't find the ad. I didn't know where it was positioned in the paper. So I looked at every ad on every page.

"I don't see it," I said. "They don't have it."

Jillian grabbed a section out of my hand and flipped it over to show it to me.

"Really?" she said.

The ad took up the entire back page of the sports section. Jillian yanked me back down the concourse to the car.

When we were at the *Today* show, it was the first time I got to watch a clip of the night before and the moment that I won, and it was unbelievable. I can't even remember the questions that the interviewer, Lester Holt, asked me; it was all such a blur. Later I saw weight loss guru Richard Simmons in the green room, and he serenaded me!

Outside on the curb, Jillian and I said good-bye. I knew, in a way, the celebration was winding up, and I'd be on to the next part of my life, and she'd be on to the next batch of contestants. I don't know how she does it. She gives so much to each person she trains. But I knew we would always stay in touch. She had teased me earlier in the season that if I won, she'd wear pink each day on camera the next season. I didn't want her to ruin her black-wearing image, but I decided to hold her to it. I bought her a necklace, like one she'd worn on the show, but in the back I had three tiny pink sapphires embedded on the clasp. She was true to her word. She e-mailed me 24 hours before she began filming the next season, frantically asking what she could wear that was pink. Coincidentally, I had just had the necklace overnighted to her that day, so she was ready to wear pink the next day, and the next. . . .

I set foot on that ranch for me, but I left that ranch for every woman, for every underdog, for everybody who'd forgotten what it felt like to dream. I swear the world wanted me to win, and I know that's the only reason I did. Once I had that idea in my head, I used that energy to push me through the moments when I wanted to give up. And whether or not people think I'm crazy for believing that, I don't really care. It doesn't mean I just put my intention out there, and that's all I did. I did do that, but I also put action behind it. I put in my workout time, I counted calories, I pushed myself. But I used every resource I had to take me to what was the biggest, most challenging goal I'd ever gone for in my life. And I knew I wasn't the only one who could do that. People everywhere can do it, too. If they believe it, they can be it.

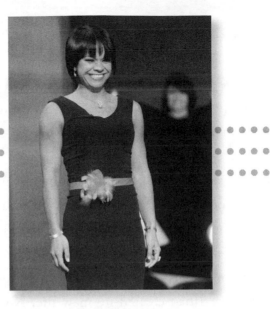

NINE

Paying It Forward

I hope I never stop dreaming and growing and going for more.

A fter wrapping up all the postfinale publicity, I arrived back home in Arizona. Now what? I knew my life was different and that I was going to take it in a different direction; I just didn't quite know what to do next. I went back to the salon and saw a few clients. I paid off my debts with my prize money—for the first time in my life, I was free of excess weight and excess debt. Of course with the prize money there were requests for help, and I gave. But I had to limit my giving in that respect, both to protect myself and because I realized that giving in that way doesn't ultimately solve anyone's problems.

Everybody seemed to have a suggestion about what I should do next, or a request that they wanted me to fulfill, and I was trying to address it all. It started to become overwhelming. I was still living at my sister Holly's house, and I knew I needed to move. I was ready to be on my own. But this time I decided to return to the place where I had created my new life. Not the ranch, of course, but the next closest thing: Los Angeles.

I thought I needed to be alone in L.A. to have new opportunities, though I didn't yet know what those opportunities would look like. So after I moved to my new place, I occupied my time by doing what I knew how to do. I would go to the gym for spin class, then swim, then do boot camp. Working out for 6 to 8 hours became working out for 8 to 10 hours. I was working out all the time. When I wasn't working out, I was sitting in my apartment or shopping for clothes. I started to do a lot of shopping. I was trading one addiction for another.

I never really settled into my apartment in L.A., because I was never there. I was always out doing something, exercising, traveling. I think I got scared because I was no longer the Ali from before *The Biggest Loser*. I felt like I needed to fill up my days with a lot of activity. I had been leading such a structured life on the ranch—secluded, sequestered, the TV people checking in all the

I Love My New Body!

I love my shoulders and my collarbone and my back. I love my shoulders because I feel like they're open and look healthy and toned. They make me want to stand proud again. I love my arms and the fact that I'm not afraid to show them anymore. I love that I don't have to think about whether something has sleeves. And I love my collarbone. It's the first bone I began feeling after I started losing weight, and I thought, "Oh my, I have a skeleton under there!"

time. And then it's all gone in a flash. Part of the reason the show is so powerful is because the people behind it give everything they have, and I appreciated their care. But they had become my number one support system, and it was hard to adjust to their absence. I thought that going back to L.A. would solve my problems, but in the end, I realized it just didn't feel right.

I had to find some balance and be okay with the calm moments in my life. I'm the kind of person who runs, runs, runs, until I pass out from exhaustion. I could either let it destroy me, or I could harness that energy and direct it toward another purpose, turn it into a blessing. I had to take the time to get focused on what I wanted to do. I believe we're all here to make a difference. I had been so focused on my problems and losing weight; now it was time to look at the bigger picture. I wanted to be a part of helping people, because I think we can create the lives we want if we just wake up and refuse to live on autopilot. But first I had to get off autopilot myself.

BELIEVE IT, BE IT FOUNDATION

While I was on the treadmill or the stairclimber, slogging through my "homework" back at the ranch, I would daydream about creating a foundation. Since King Gillette Ranch, where *The Biggest Loser* is taped, is also a state park, there were nature camps and forest rangers taking kids on hikes all around us. Sometimes we'd run into them, and toward the end the kids would come up and ask me to sign autographs. They said they were proud of me. I told the kids that a lot of the exercises we did on the ranch were the same ones I learned in phys ed class when I was a kid, like squats and lunges and pushups, that kind of thing. And a lot of them said that their schools didn't offer phys ed anymore. I was shocked when I learned that many public schools were eliminating gym classes because of budget cuts. I think that learning about exercise and nutrition is just as important as academics for kids. And playing sports is important, too—you learn how to be on a team, how to push yourself and achieve goals. So sometimes when I was on the treadmill, I'd think to myself, "That's what I want to do. I'm going to start a foundation to help these kids get healthy."

When I considered it, I decided I wanted to create a program open to all kids, but one that would especially benefit young girls. I wanted them to learn to feel good about themselves in a supportive social environment where they would receive encourage-ment and develop confidence. Why not teach kids all those things through health and fitness? In a country increasingly threatened by rising childhood obesity and type 2 diabetes, why not teach them that 3,500 calories equals 1 pound—something I never learned until much later in life? And, most important, I wanted every child to one day know what it's like to experience a moment of pride and success in their lives, like the moment I had when I stood up on the scale at *The Biggest Loser* finale.

I took my 13-year-old niece, Alexis, with me to New York City when I went there for a photo shoot with *Prevention* maga-zine in 2008. After the shoot, we were sitting in a restaurant chat-ting, and I asked her about her dreams and goals for the future.

"I'm just not really good at anything," she said.

"What do you mean?" I asked her.

"I'm just a middle-of-the-road girl," she said. "I like to follow rules."

I remembered Alexis sharing a story earlier that day as we walked around the city about how she loved following the rules at school. She didn't see how liking to follow rules could help her stand out in any way. But rules, I told her, needed to be followed in lots of situations, like student government, for example. "I didn't think of it that way," she said. She said she also wanted to go to New York University one day, but her initial thought was "There's no way." Of course there's a way!

That's what I want the Believe It, Be It Foundation to be all about—helping kids find whatever it is that makes them feel good about themselves, showing them ways they can follow their dreams. It will be rooted in health and wellness and will help draw out and celebrate every child's innate gifts and aspirations. I know it will include sports in some way, as I think sports help girls develop confidence and learn how to compete against one another in a healthy way. I want to create a sorority of girls that will eventually stretch across generations.

I still have no idea exactly how we'll get there. But I know we will. I'll get there. And that's a huge departure from how I was thinking about life just a year ago. I've set a new goal, and I know that it will help guide me through the next phase of my life.

IN THE MEANTIME

I called a meeting (which was a first for me, "calling a meeting") with Mark Koops, the managing director of Reveille, which is the production company that produces *The Biggest Loser*. And he accepted! When we met, I told him that *The Biggest Loser* had helped me find myself and regain control of my life. I had been receiving e-mails saying, "Thank you for changing the consciousness of America." I wanted to keep being a part of that. I wanted to connect with regular girls like me, regular moms, regular young women, and reassure them that if they were headed in a direction they didn't want to go, they could change that. They just had to make a choice.

Mark told me that he'd been waiting for this meeting for 5

years, waiting for a woman to walk through the door who wanted to be a part of making a difference. So, working with *The Biggest Loser* and sponsors such as 24 Hour Fitness and Designer Whey protein powder, I've been able to get out and speak at events and build relationships with amazing women all over the country— women who have been watching the world go by for too long, wanting to change but not believing that they can. I want to give them the tools and motivation that were given to me, and help them realize their dreams.

WHAT LOVE HAS TO DO WITH IT

I know that lots of people come to hear me talk thinking I'm going to delve deep into weight loss strategies—but that's not why I do what I do; that's not my big-picture focus. What I'm passionate about is finally believing in myself again. I want to share my journey of falling in love with myself. Because *love* is the one word people don't usually associate with weight loss.

I think that one of the reasons I make connections with people so easily is because I'm just a normal person who went through an extraordinary journey—one that happened to be on national television. But the important thing I want people to understand is that they deserve to have what I have, too—they deserve to have their best possible lives. I want to lead by example, and I'm an example of what it looks like to believe in yourself.

I especially like to focus on helping women, who often are living so short of their full potential, and a lot of times that's because extra weight is holding them back from feeling good about themselves. The number one culprit I see in that equation is the lack of time women allow themselves to get healthy and stay healthy. When did it become okay to give your time to everyone but yourself? Women tend to nurture on so many different levels for so many people that they often forget to take care of themselves.

It's so important to check in with yourself, no matter how busy you are—to ask yourself what you need in order to live a happy life. Finding the time for exercise can be a challenge, but you can start with small steps—finding ways to incorporate more activity into your day. You don't have to go to the gym. You can ride bikes with your husband in the morning before work, take your dog for a walk, run the perimeter of the soccer field while your kids are at practice.

I love talking to people and being a part of their lives. I used to tremble if I had to speak in front of a handful of people. Now I can talk to an audience of 2,000 without feeling any nerves! That's because I believe talking to people is important. I want to

• •

PLAN—AND DON'T GET DERAILED!

I *always* have snacks with me so that I'm always prepared if the day gets away from me and I find myself getting hungry. I carry almonds, fruit, string cheese, or packets of protein powder that I can mix with water.

• •

Do It Your Way

Celebrations don't always have to be about food. Try celebrating important occasions in other ways. For example, on my birthday, I want to go to a group spin class. Instead of being in a restaurant and feeling tempted, I want all my friends to come and sweat with me! For you it might be a day of swimming at the beach with your kids or a tango lesson with your husband. There are lots of ways to celebrate without calories.

establish a connection with each and every person in that audience, because I know they can relate to my struggle.

I hear stories from all walks of life. So many women are struggling to build healthy relationships with their mothers, their sisters, their friends, their spouses. They have to find ways to communicate their needs to these very important people in their lives. And I don't have all the answers. But I can listen, and I can relate what I've learned on my journey. That's what I have to give.

DAY AFTER DAY

Big, sweeping life changes really boil down to small, everyday decisions. I know counting calories can be a chore, but if I don't count them, how am I going to know how many I put in my body? I want to stay aware; I don't want to put my head in the sand because

I'm afraid to know how much I'm eating. Counting calories puts me in control. You have to find a good, healthy balance, though. Don't let your vigilance keep you from enjoying the foods you love—use it to help you enjoy those foods in moderation.

The same principle is true with exercise. Sometimes there are just days when I don't want to get on the treadmill. But I love the results when I do. I love how I feel after I've exercised—it gives me energy for the rest of the day. Take ownership of what exercise accomplishes for you, how it moves you closer to your goal of feeling good, healthy, and strong. It's important to own whatever activity you engage in and give it your best effort. When I swept the floors at the beauty salon, I loved that my area was spotless. I got burns on my arms from making perfect pizzas. I loved being the best at even those simple tasks. It gives me a sense of pride and accomplishment to do something well, even if I don't always enjoy the task at hand.

Resistance is never the agent of change. You have to embrace the actions that are going to get you closer to your goal. Praise yourself for meeting each challenge on the way to that goal. You're going to have to buckle down and do some hard work—but think of where it's going to take you!

Remember, when weight loss becomes a goal in your life, eating right and exercising are just two pieces of the puzzle. Figuring out why you've put on the extra weight is the hardest part. Asking yourself why you've made some poor choices, what kinds of feelings you might have been trying to avoid—it's not easy. But you

• •

FEELING STUCK?

You can either change what's making you feel stuck or change the way you think about it. Let's say you have a job you don't like, but you need it to pay your bills. Then learn to love the "why" of the job. You're supporting your family, which is a blessing! Find the positive in tough situations. Thinking this way is going to get you out of ruts. Collect evidence for the success in a situation.

• •

have to dive into that emotional part of it. Because how you feel about yourself is reflected in your body. I believe that my body is a direct reflection of how I feel now, and I also know it was a direct reflection of how I felt at 234 pounds.

It's so important to have trusting, supportive relationships when you're going through this process. You need to be able to share your feelings with people who will help you really dig deeper and figure out what's going on inside. I think so many of us have gotten used to putting ourselves on the back burner that it's been years—as it was in my case—since we've really told the truth about who we want to be in this world, what kinds of things we want for ourselves. Finding people you can talk to, who will listen to you and advise you without judgment, is key.

I hug a lot of the people I meet. I've probably hugged thousands of people at this point. Sometimes when I'm in an airport, total strangers will run up to me and hug me, and I hug them right back—because everyone needs to feel like they are valued and appreciated. Everyone deserves a hug! When I hug these people, I am wishing the best for them. I'm thinking, "You can do it." I just hope that they can learn to believe it—and be it—for themselves.

MAINTENANCE

I thought maintenance was going to be a lot harder than it has ended up being. You work your tail off to get to a certain point, and then it becomes about living your life and being mindful of your choices. You don't have to be in the gym a million hours a day. You don't have to completely avoid all the foods you love. You just have to find a balance. Yes, you do have to watch your calories, and you do have to put in those hours in the gym, but once you've developed a healthy lifestyle and changed your values and priorities, it just fits.

Maintenance is about finding a balance and figuring out what you need to do to stay where you want to be. I still keep a food journal in my handbag! That's the reality. This is the rest of my life. I want to feel healthy and happy every day for the rest of my life, and the only way to take control of that is to keep doing what I'm doing.

ALL IN THE FAMILY

In the year since I won *The Biggest Loser,* my relationship with my mom has been the best that we've ever experienced. It feels health-

• •

I LOVE BEING ACTIVE

These days I spend about 2 hours in the gym a minimum of 5 days a week. I usually try to do 6 days a week, with 1 day off always. I work out with a trainer 3 days a week, but I train with weights and resistance machines 5 days a week. For cardio, I like the stair-climber. It's a good way for me to work up a sweat. Once I'm covered in sweat, I know I've done my job.

• •

ier, and there's less tension. We are both much happier people now, which makes it easier to get along. That doesn't mean we don't have our ups and downs. But I've learned how to ask for her support. And I know how to dig my way out of sticky mother-daughter conflicts much more quickly than before, when our fights would sometimes drag on for weeks.

My mom is still working toward her weight loss goal, but she's had to undergo surgeries on her knee and both of her hands, so she's been avoiding the gym. Her challenge is to find ways to exercise around her injuries. She can swim and work out on a recumbent bike, for example, but it's a challenge for her mentally to get back into it. Sometimes she's able to, but other times I think she just finds the prospect of exercising with an injured body too overwhelming. But even with all these challenges, she's kept off the weight she lost on the ranch and even lost some more! I am proud of her every day.

I think when I lost so much weight and won *The Biggest Loser,* our roles shifted a little bit. Mom has always been the one who got all the attention; she enjoys being in the spotlight. Now, when we're out in public together, if I'm recognized and she's not, she's quick to remind people who she is. On the other hand, if we're out together and neither one of us is recognized, she's quick to point out to everyone who I am!

Like lots of other women, Mom tends to invalidate herself sometimes, saying, "I'm no Buba," in terms of her weight loss progress. That's when I have to say, "Mom, why do you keep comparing yourself to me? Do I need to carry around a picture of you to constantly remind you of your success?" I try to acknowledge and remind her of the amazing things she's already accomplished. The real reward will be seeing her recognize that and pat herself on the back one day.

And after watching her daughter and her granddaughter get in shape, my grandma has also been inspired to become more active. She's started walking to the mailbox every day and is just

• •

WORK AROUND INJURIES

Sometimes we can let injuries scare us away from exercise. But there's always something you can do if you're just willing to look for it. Find ways to keep moving. The longer you put it off, the harder it's going to be to walk through those gym doors again.

• •

moving around more. She's thinking about her health differently. She even got a Bodybugg! (Maybe I should decorate hers with pink crystals, like I did mine!)

It's nice to feel like I am contributing to my family in ways I was never able to before, from hiking and going on bike rides to cooking a healthy dinner and hanging around the table talking— not eating seconds and thirds. I'm not shut down and cut off from the ones I love anymore, because I'm no longer ashamed of the choices I make.

A Conversation with Alexis

When I was competing on *The Biggest Loser* and it was clear that I had a shot at winning, Jillian and I strategized about what number on the scale would get me there. As long as it was healthy for my height, I was good with it. I knew I would have to push really hard to make that number. I'd have to train intensely, like an athlete. And I would be judged on those efforts by stepping up on the scale each week. I was fine with that. But knowing that my nieces and nephew would be watching, I wanted them to understand what success really meant to me. Yes, I wanted to win, and I was competing to win. But the most important part of this process was getting my life back and becoming healthier, stronger, and more confident and energetic. I wanted them to understand that it wasn't just about a number on a scale.

My weight was a common topic of conversation in my family, so I felt it was especially important to talk to my 13-year-old niece, Alexis, about body image and weight loss. I wanted to make sure that she understood what the process I was undergoing was all about. I had always been the overweight aunt, and now I wasn't. Alexis was even being teased by her little brother, McCoy, in true little brother fashion, that soon I would weigh less than she did. When I heard this, I knew I needed to talk to her. I wanted her to know three things: First, there was no way I would ever weigh the same as her, let alone less! Second, when I left the ranch to train for the finale, I was already healthy—I was only losing more weight and training like an athlete to win the competition. And third, no matter what number appeared on that scale at the finale, she needed to know I had already won, because I had won my life back! Kids are extremely perceptive and pick up a lot of what is going on around them, so it's our job to ensure that they correctly understand the information they're exposed to.

My oldest niece, Alex (McCoy and Alexis's older sister), is a star athlete, and her college soccer team won the national title in their division. When I arrived home after being eliminated from the ranch, Alex was in Arizona for soccer and decided she was going to work out with me, so we ran drills on the treadmill. She couldn't believe it. Here was her aunt, the one who used to always look for a chair, running right along next to her! I was always the aunt with the cool handbags and makeup, but now I'm also the aunt with the great-fitting designer jeans. It felt so good to be the new Aunt Ali who was confident and proud of herself—and who could relate to the healthy young woman Alex is in a whole new way. Alex and her friends even started borrowing some of my clothes!

It's just so important for me to acknowledge the role my family has played throughout my weight loss—the family I avoided all those years. Everyone has pitched in at one point or another to support me, from Mom being on the show with me, to my sisters helping me in every possible way, to my grandma's love, to my brothers' cross-training drills, to my nieces and nephews and step-mom biking with me—even my dad came to a spin class with me! Everybody made choices to support my choices. And I will never stop feeling that love and drawing from it.

And, I've fallen in love! Before, I tested relationships way too early, panicked that I might not really be loved—I always needed to have reassurance from the get-go. I always wanted to find out quickly whether a relationship was going to be "forever"—not a great way to let love grow. But now I've met the most amazing person, who just wants me to be happy, to do what makes me happy. I used to feel I had to earn love. Now I can just be me. And I don't need to constantly check in. I'm not afraid of being left anymore. Being comfortable with myself, finding balance, taking care of myself—it's liberation in the truest sense.

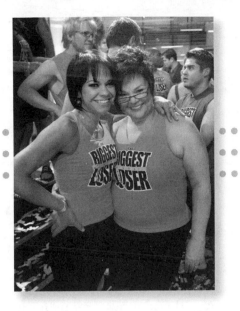

TEN

How to Believe It, Be It

Today I feel beautiful, I feel strong, I feel confident. Beauty is about feeling good, and it's about going after what you want and believing in yourself. That's what is going to make you fall in love with your life again. I can do and be and have everything I want in life. And so can you.

BELIEVE IN YOURSELF—AGAIN OR FOR THE FIRST TIME IN YOUR LIFE

If you want to make big and lasting changes, especially from a weight loss perspective, the first person you need to get on board is you. When we're feeling stuck, not living the lives we were meant to live, not feeling the love and happiness and connection we all deserve to have, it usually means we've lost faith in ourselves.

During those dark years when I was overweight and unhappy, I was always on edge. I was always waiting for someone to attack me, to criticize or judge me. What I realized later is that I was the one doing the judging. I was the one who was putting myself in a box. The liberating part of my journey was the realization that if I could put myself in there, I also had the power to let myself out. I held the key to that box.

The bottom line was that I had to accept me. I had to love me. I had to know that I was worthy of having what I wanted in life. It was just knowing that I'm worth what I want for myself. I was the one making myself feel excluded from my family, because I wasn't showing up, I wasn't talking, I wasn't sharing. I didn't have a lot of depth in my relationships, because I didn't feel like I could be honest, that I could expose who I really was.

Part of the problem was that I wasn't proud of myself. I wasn't proud of the fact that I wasn't doing anything to contribute to my family or my community. I was just existing. It's hard to admit to yourself or anyone else that you don't love yourself. But in the process of losing and letting go of my weight—my protection from the world—I needed to tell the truth. I looked at my past and my present and acknowledged the times in my life that I was really proud of, and the times that I wasn't. I had to do that to turn things around. I had to become active in my community. I had to start calling my friends again and being willing to put myself in front of new people and participate in conversations. I was supposed to be visible, just like anyone else.

Learning to love yourself isn't easy. At first, you may not feel like you can do it, but you have to try. Nurture your body with wholesome food, fresh air, exercise, and enough rest. Follow your

• •

MUSCLE MASS

As women, we're hesitant to build our bodies because we don't want to look big and burly. But building strength is important. In order for me to lose as much hydrated fat as I needed to, I had to build lean muscle mass, which eats up fat at a faster rate. You're not going to get bulky, especially if you do your cardio. I know that my body genetically has a tendency to bulk up, but I do so much cardio that it counteracts it. Remember when my goal was to wear sleeveless shirts? Have you seen me in anything *but* since *The Biggest Loser*?

• •

program for healthy living and learn what that takes. And start showing up for life. You have so much to offer. Pretty soon, you'll become more and more proactive about your destiny, because you'll have the energy and confidence to make your dreams your reality.

DIG DEEP

When I meet people and they ask me how I lost the weight and how *they* can lose the weight, I tell them first you need to figure out where are you right now—physically, emotionally, mentally, and spiritually. And you need to be honest.

I went on national TV and dug into the hardest, most personal questions I can imagine: "Why do I overeat? Why do I punish myself? Why am I unhappy?" The answer to all three questions, I discovered, was the same: Because I wasn't willing to look at my life and deal with it. I wasn't able to admit that I didn't have any goals for my future. I wasn't able to admit that I wasn't in a relationship and I really just wanted to love and be loved. I wasn't able to admit that I was settling in my career because I didn't have the confidence to take it to the next level.

Once you understand where you've been, you can start to figure out where you want to go. Start picturing what you want your future to look like—and I'm not talking about after you've lost the weight. I mean, what types of relationships would you create? How would you contribute to your community? How would you continue to challenge yourself physically? And at work? You need

(continued on page 144)

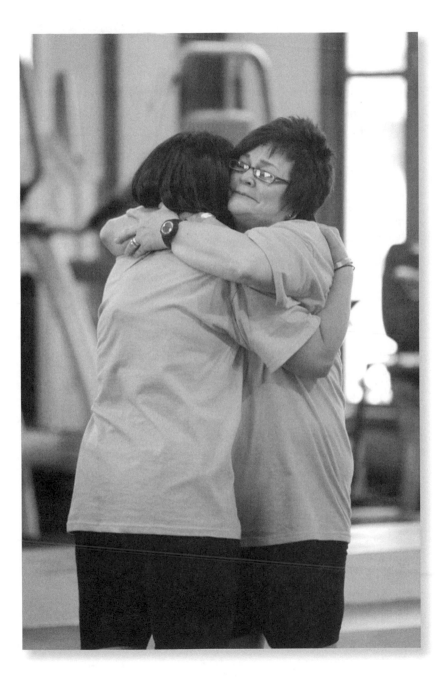

MY BUCKET LIST

There are no better tools for accountability than pen and paper. When we first arrived at the ranch, Jillian asked us to make two lists. The first one was in response to the question, "Why are you here in the first place? What brought you to this point?" The second was "What do you want in life?"

Here's what I wrote down. I kept these lists long after this task at the ranch and still refer to them to remind me of where I came from and where I'm going. I find them helpful and recommend that you do the same.

WHY I AM HERE

I've always felt alone.

Protection.

When I feel lonely, I eat to try and fulfill the emptiness inside.

It's my shelter.

My excuse.

Makes me "right"

It's my security.

I quit playing the game. Love me the way I am or don't love me at all. (Then I'll show them and lose weight.)

I thought I met the person I would share my life with. Within a year my grandfather died (my safety net); my relationship ended (and I had given up a career in San Francisco, planning to move to Indonesia to be with this person); my dog of 10 years died. I gained back the weight I started to lose plus 60 pounds.

WHAT I WANT

To be happy

To be in a loving, lasting relationship

To have a baby

To be successful in my career

To travel the world

To be healthy

To live a long life

To be a role model

To dance

To learn to sing

To be debt-free

To have a fashionable wardrobe

To have continuous joy

To trust

To embrace peace and spirituality

To be accepted

To have good posture

To enjoy running

To do a triathlon

To raise a healthy happy child

To accept and trust love

To give to my community

To take time to enjoy the arts

To love

to know where you are and what you want before you can create a productive, happy future.

When I was overweight and unhappy, I *thought* about being smaller, I *thought* about fitting into different clothes and feeling comfortable in any environment or social situation. But I didn't *do* anything about it. I was letting myself fall victim to not planning, not clarifying steps to reach my goals. Don't go on just wanting something. Start consciously planning where you want to be.

NEVER STOP FACING YOUR FEARS

As contestants on *The Biggest Loser,* we had our fears constantly put to the test each week through the physical challenges we endured. But you don't have to be on TV to let life scare you. The important thing is to not let it stop you. Letting fear have its way will prevent you from having everything you ever wanted. There is tremendous power in recognizing the fear in something and doing it anyway. "Do it scared," as the old saying goes.

Have you ever seen those T-shirts that say, "NO FEAR"? Well, my mom used to say they should read, "KNOW FEAR," because *that's* how you make dreams happen. When you have the courage to tell the truth about what you're really afraid of, fear doesn't have control over your life.

I wasn't ever afraid of working hard in the gym and spending all the time it took to prepare and track my calories, or having to decline certain invitations that didn't support my weight loss efforts. But I was afraid that if I actually reached my goal weight and all the things that I wanted in my life still didn't happen, it would mean that there was something wrong with me, that I was never going to have what I wanted. My weight, which had protected me for so long, wouldn't be an excuse anymore.

CREATE YOUR OWN DESTINY

It breaks my heart when I hear people say, "Oh, I've tried out for *The Biggest Loser* for four seasons in a row, and I'm trying out again." If you're big enough to try out for *The Biggest Loser,* you know you have not just a weight problem, but a health problem. When you stand in that line, you have acknowledged that it's time to make changes in your life, whether or not you are lucky enough to make it onto the show. The minute I stood in line with my mom, I knew the gig was up. No matter what, I had to figure out a way to make a change and lose the weight. I was just trying to find the right path to help me do it. If *The Biggest Loser* didn't turn out to be that path, I was going to find another.

Nine months before we went to *The Biggest Loser* ranch, my mom was at the hospital, undergoing an angiogram when her heart suddenly stopped beating. The doctors resuscitated her, and she survived on life support for the next 48 hours. When she woke up, in complete Bette-Sue fashion, she thought everything was fine. But Amber and I were shaken to our core. We thought we had lost our mother. We knew it was time to get healthy—we had no choice.

This is your life and your health at stake, so don't wait for a casting director's decision to determine your destiny. Use your passion for the show as motivation and inspiration—not as an excuse to put off the changes you need to make.

Sometimes people say, "Oh, I could lose the weight, too, if I could go to *The Biggest Loser* ranch." It's true that it's easier to stick to a program when you're constantly being monitored and you don't have to contend with the daily distractions of your environment at home. But even for contestants at the ranch, you can only be watched so much. If you can't stay true to your goals when nobody is watching, then you will never be successful in the long run. These days, when I visit the ranch, I want to take every single contestant in my arms and reassure them that everything will be okay—the competition, the alliances, the eliminations— none of it really matters. Whether they stay on the ranch or go home, the important thing is finding a way to make lasting changes. For contestants on *The Biggest Loser,* time on the ranch is special, but in the bigger picture, it's just a fleeting moment of our lives. Being on the show is a privilege and a blessing, but it doesn't guarantee success in the long run. You have to create that for yourself. *The Biggest Loser* gives you the tools, but each individual has to choose to use them every single day, to create their own long-term success.

• •

AFTER-DINNER SNACKING

If you have a problem with snacking after dinner, the best advice is just to acknowledge what your pattern is. If you know you're going to think about food after dinner, then make sure you budget to have a snack after dinner. It doesn't really matter when you have your snacks, as long as you allow for the calories in your daily allotment.

• •

FORGIVE YOURSELF

Look, I'm not perfect. Everybody slips, particularly with calorie budgets. We're used to turning to food for comfort, so sometimes we may find ourselves reaching for a cookie or grabbing a slice of pizza we didn't budget for. Just don't take it to the next day. Wake up the next morning, go to the gym, and put it behind you. Keep moving forward. Beating yourself up is just going to send you right back to that old place where you used to hang out. To avoid triggers, it's a good idea to write down everything you eat. I still do. Stay aware of your choices and why you're making them. Don't try to pretend they might not show up on the scale. Just understand your results so you can make better choices next time.

The important thing is to remember that this is a process; it's not about perfection. Health and happiness are about being in the moment, recognizing old patterns and being aware of them. I have to work at making the right choices every day. The difference now is that I don't let one slipup ruin a whole day, or a week, or a month. Just stay aware. Talk to friends. Journal. Find support online. Don't bury your feelings.

Sometimes you'll be hit out of the blue with feelings of inadequacy, of not being appreciated, of not feeling worthy. Are you worthy? Are you kidding me? Of course you're worthy! Those are old feelings, how you felt in the past. But now you're acknowledging them and making different choices about how to handle them. And eating won't solve anything. Try making different choices. Get in the car and go to the gym, even if you just sit in the parking lot. Okay, now you're in the parking lot. Why don't you just go in for 15 minutes? You can sit in the locker room for a while if you want. Then maybe you can walk on the treadmill for a few minutes. You're going to get past those old, bad feelings. Just acknowledge them, be okay with them, and keep moving forward, inch by inch.

Being resistant is not being proactive. I have to choose my healthy lifestyle every day. Some days it's one moment at a time. I can stop and break down my obstacles and figure out the steps to overcoming them. Break challenges down into small steps, as you would any other obstacle in your life. So I come home after traveling and working long days and my house is a disaster? Okay, I'll start by unpacking my bags. Then I can sort the laundry. I can start to feel a little less overwhelmed, and I can choose to feel good in the next moment. And the next. When you're happy with yourself, you can make healthier, more productive choices.

EMBRACE THE GREATNESS WITHIN

Each season of *The Biggest Loser,* I watch contestants move from a place of fear and hurt and feeling small to confidence and joy and bounty in their newfound selves. But the thing is, the possibility for greatness was always within each and every one of them.

They just had to make the decision to let it emerge. That's why the end of each season is always such a joy, to see the contestants realize that that inner greatness has come out and shone for the whole world to witness. Who can forget watching Helen Phillips run that 26th mile in her season's final challenge and yell to everyone on the beach as she approached the finish line: "Look at me! I'm a marathon runner!" I was stationed at mile 13 to meet and encourage the final four contestants—Helen, Tara Costa, Ron Morelli, and Mike Morelli—for that final and amazing challenge, all 26.2 miles. As I stood there waiting, I kept thinking that not only were they running a marathon, they were running a marathon with *hills!* "Shoot," I thought, thinking like an Arizona girl, "they didn't even get to run a *flat* marathon."

Tara was the first to arrive, and she was so on her pace, I couldn't even stop her to give her a hug! We ran together for about a mile, and I told her how proud of her I was. She was on track to do this marathon in less than 5 hours. Then I jogged back to mile

• •

APPRECIATE OTHERS

Now that I'm fit, I love looking at people—admiring their arms or body tone. It's not a judgmental thing. It's just that when I was over-weight, I was so unhappy with my body that I basically never looked at anyone else. Practice being aware not only of yourself but of others' presence. It's a way to stay conscious and connected to them.

• •

13 to find Helen approaching, and she was exultant. "I'm doing this!" she said. Then Mike came later, walking due to a hip injury but not giving up because of it. Hours later, there was his dad, Ron, with bad knees, bad shoulders, and a cane. Other former contestants, including Bernie Salazar, Jim Germanakos, Heba Salama, and Michelle Aguilar, joined me in walking with Ron the remaining miles. I knew Ron was struggling, but I also knew he wasn't going to stop.

It's such a pleasure to see other *Biggest Loser* alumni living the lives they've always wanted after being on the show. There's Dan Evans out there singing and touring and making his name in the music world. Curtis and Mallory Bray are now personal trainers, setting a great example for their young girls. Mark Kruger is now a weekend spin instructor, and despite being teased about all the emotion that poured out of him at the ranch, he's closer to his kids and family than ever. He's not holding back anymore. Bernie Salazar recently ran in the Chicago Marathon and is working on a children's book. You just can't help but be changed by the experience.

At the ranch, I began the journey of my life, the biggest thing I have ever done to date. And it didn't start with the workouts or the eating, but with embracing the belief that I had something great within me. There's always been a light inside me that I just let dim over the years through the layers of fat. But it never went out. When I was on the treadmill at the ranch, I started fanning that flame again and it grew, just as my family and friends fanned it with their support. That light just caught fire! I never want to live with my light on dim ever again.

I learned that when Michelangelo was asked how he could carve something as beautiful as the figure of David out of stone, he is thought to have said that he studied the plain slab of marble until he saw the figure within and just carved away the excess until David

• •

LEARNING TO CHOOSE

You know how hard it was for me to make it to that finale. You know about my struggles. Has it gotten any easier? Not always. It's just about making the right choices over and over. What is easier is that I can make the right choices a little quicker than I used to. But I have to remember that for 30 years, I ate a certain way. I have to remember each day to do the right thing for my body and my health. This is for the rest of my life.

• •

emerged. That's how I want everyone to feel. I want them to see the possibility within themselves. I want them to find their David.

ACKNOWLEDGE YOUR PHYSICAL STRENGTH AND ENDURANCE

Physical challenges are also mental challenges. At the ranch, contestants discover over and over that they can do far more than they realize, that their limitations are often self-imposed. I felt mentally and physically depleted at times, but those feelings became something I knew I could overcome. And now, knowing what I was able to endure serves as inspiration for me when I need strength.

I still try to do things that push my limits. Camelback Mountain in Phoenix is one of the biggest mountains in the area where I live. For years, I'd heard everybody talk about how hard it was to hike. I was afraid of hiking. I didn't really know what it meant, what it entailed.

But after *The Biggest Loser,* I thought, "What's stopping me? Let's just do this." I drove to the mountain with some friends, and we had to wait in line to park—the parking lot was jammed. There was an immediate excuse. I was ready to just give up and go home.

But I didn't turn around. We waited in line, parked, and then I literally put one foot in front of the other and started hiking that mountain. As it turned out, there were lots of different people hiking, of all shapes and sizes and ages. Some were running and some were not. It was challenging, but I could do it. I felt good. All of that fear was for nothing.

It's the same with weight loss. When you think about having to lose 100 pounds, it feels like you have to climb Camelback Mountain. "There's no way," you think to yourself. But you can do it if you just break it down and take it one step at a time.

When I stood at the top of that mountain, I felt the power from climbing it. It was something I had denied myself in the past, because I'd felt it was impossible; I'd felt afraid of it. I had let my fear of my abilities stop me from even trying.

I watched a documentary recently about the Ironman Triathlon, which consists of a 2.4-mile swim, a 112-mile bike ride, and a full (26.2-mile) marathon—raced in that order and without a break! Honestly, watching competitors in that triathlon echoed how I felt competing on *The Biggest Loser*. Like those athletes, I chose to compete in incredibly tough conditions. And it paid off in volumes for my soul and spirit. So find something that will give you that experience. Something that you're scared of. Let the possibility of accomplishment blossom within you.

COLLECT EVIDENCE FOR SUCCESS

Carrying around a lot of excess weight can definitely act as a negative filter to our thinking. And, like dominoes, those negative thoughts can lead to more negative consequences. You have to turn around that pattern around before it dominates your whole outlook.

When Mom and I were sent home at the end of the fourth week, I could have thought, "What's the point? I'll never be the Biggest Loser," and thrown in the towel. I had no idea I was going to get a second chance. But when I went home, I decided I would become the unofficial Biggest Loser, if not the one who wins the grand prize. I'd still work hard and come back to the finale with the biggest weight loss percentage of all. I had no idea I'd have the opportunity to go back to the ranch and vie for the big title. Approaching the next weeks that way meant that when the phone call came to come back to the ranch, I really was in the position to win a place back at the ranch and become the Biggest Loser.

But the point is, I was going to succeed, whether that call came through or not. So stop seeing the obstacles you face as reasons why you can't do something. See them as a reason why you can. And celebrate your accomplishments on a daily basis. I celebrated every pound I lost. Since I beat myself up for gaining them, I was going to feel good about losing them!

There are so many fun ways to build the habit of collecting evidence for success. Remember that Mom and I stood in line to be cast in the show on the 11th day of the month and were the 11th pair in line. We decided to take that as a good sign! Our season was the first that had teams, and we were the first mother-daughter team. Yay! Our color was pink, the color often associated with strong women who are fighters. We'll take it! I started to notice pink everywhere . . . pink in store windows when I was home, pink in flowers, and pink in the sky. When I was training for the finale at the gym, I even noticed ladies wearing workout pants from Victoria's Secret with "Team Pink" written across their behinds. Every time I saw them, I felt like they were rooting for me and my success. I collected evidence that I was going to be the first female Biggest Loser, and I created it. Does it matter that I wore a pink shirt? No. Does pink inherently have power? No. But if I say pink has power, if I believe that, it does! At the end of the day, it's just a T-shirt. But my belief made it so much more than that.

COMMUNICATE YOUR NEEDS

When I was overweight, I thought that my family judged me. They would try to help me with my diet and exercise, and I knew they wanted to be supportive, but it felt like judgment. I felt they were being the food police, which made me want to pull away from them. That was one of the hardest things about coming home: I needed to figure out a way to communicate how I needed to be supported.

When you're making a big change in your life, sometimes you have to sit down with the people you love and have hard conversations. The truth is that most of the time they just want to support you, but they probably don't know the best way to do that—so you need to tell them. You want to be able to live your life around the people you love. In my case, I needed to be honest and say, "I want your help, I need your help—but I don't want you to police me. I want you to be there for me without trying to control me. I want you to listen to me without having all the answers or telling me what's right or wrong. Just listen."

Once a woman I was talking with told me that she felt as if her husband was always watching what she ate. This is such a common situation for overweight people—feeling judged by those around them when they eat. When you feel scrutinized like that, you start sneaking food. You eat in secret to avoid other people's stares. You're not out in the open, and it feels disgusting and wrong. The act of eating is about nourishing your body—it should never feel like that.

Let's say someone in your support group notices you snacking and knows you just had lunch. Instead of saying, "Are you sure you want to eat that?" or "Oh, don't you think that's a lot? You just ate . . . ," ask them to try distracting you, not policing you. They can say, "Hey, let's go shopping" or "Let's go to a movie." Offer an alternative to saying something that feels accusatory. There are so many broken relationships around people struggling with their weight, because they're not able to communicate what actions will feel like support.

GIVE BACK AND HELP OTHERS FIND THEIR DREAMS

I'm a great believer in the power of community, of spreading the good energy we get from accomplishing our goals, of becoming better people and empowering others to do the same. I love shar-

• •

LISTEN TO YOUR BODY

If there's a day when I wake up and I'm really tired, I check in with myself. What's going on here? Am I stressed or overwhelmed about something? Do I need to take a break? Maybe I just need a day off. If that's the case, I rest. But if it happens day after day, something else is going on in my life, and I have to pay attention to that. I have to figure out what's not working.

• •

ing with people, and I do it all the time. In airports, walking down the street—people stop me and we talk. I love connecting with people. I want to have a world of girlfriends!

There are so many ways to give back. For me, it's meeting and talking with people all across the country and working on my Believe It, Be It Foundation. When you've been able to achieve your own goals, you have the power to help other people figure out what their dreams are, show them how to take the steps. And I think that's how we stay alive and in the moment, aware. That's the epitome of health—openness and connection. Maybe there's a service project in your community you want to be a part of—a toy drive, a school fund-raiser, a neighborhood cleanup, whatever. If it's a project that's positive in nature, then it's helping to create a healthy community.

For 10 years, I felt I didn't make a difference in anyone's life; I was holding myself back. My smiles weren't sincere. I was living smaller than I knew I wanted to live. I felt bad about myself and removed myself from life. It wasn't a constant low, but there were lots of lows. In so many ways, I was settling. I was scared of being turned down. I didn't even know what I was capable of doing.

TALK TO YOURSELF!

Every time I exercise, I have a conversation with myself. Why? Because I don't do stuff that I'm comfortable doing. If I'm comfortable, then it's not doing anything for me, and I don't consider it working out. If I'm just going for a walk, that's fine. That's activity, and it's good. But to push myself, I'll go running. And it doesn't matter what the run is, I usually end up wanting to quit in the middle. It's a mental thing for me, and I have to say, "Okay, Ali, you don't really want to give up. You only want to give up because you're feeling uncomfortable."

I have a physically strong body that I built and that will endure and will perform at a demanding level. But every day when I work out, I come up against the limits of my mind. I have to trick myself sometimes. If I'm running and want to stop, I just say, "Okay, just run to that tree. You can quit there." But often I'm willing to push myself just a little more. So I say, "Okay, I can make it to the next tree that's 10 yards away." And the next thing I know I'm halfway to the finish line! And when I run the distance I had set out to run, I have such a feeling of accomplishment. That's how you build confidence in yourself.

I do the same thing with food. If I find myself mindlessly

snacking, I'll sometimes stop and think, "Am I really hungry, or am I tired?" I go, go, go so much, I sometimes have to let myself slow down and think about my energy level. I don't keep tempting stuff in my kitchen—I childproof my house in that way. But I don't want to practice mindless eating, even if it's healthy foods like grapes or almonds. Often, I just need to turn off the TV and go to bed. Sometimes I just have to tell myself it's time to rest.

LET FRIENDSHIPS EVOLVE

When you lose weight, sometimes friends can feel threatened or off balance. You've changed the equation of your relationship, and some friends may want things to go back to the way they used to be. Maybe you used to go eat pizza together or go out partying all the time. You've played a certain role in their lives, and while they may be excited for you, they also may be afraid of losing the relationship they are accustomed to having with you.

Be honest with them. If they invite you into old environments that you no longer feel comfortable being in, places where you're tempted to overeat or do activities that don't support your healthy lifestyle, tell them that you love them but you can't spend time with them in the same way you used to. You still value their friendship, but you also need to stay true to your goals. Suggest something else, a place where you can eat a healthy meal or, even better, a physical activity you might enjoy together. You can change the old patterns, and make new ones. And if your friend isn't willing to adapt, it may not be a friendship that's meant to last.

Remember, you are now building a world that works for you, that reflects your beliefs, and that nurtures your healthy self— your best self. Making sure this world and your relationships reflect your new life of conscious decisions will keep you on a true course to realizing your goals.

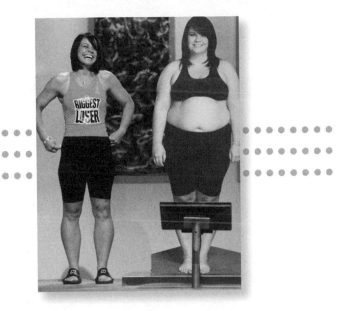

Closing Thoughts

As I reflect on all that I've shared in this book, I want to add a couple of important thoughts.

After I gave a speech on the road recently, a man approached me and asked, "If you carried around all that extra weight for protection, what's protecting you now?" I thought that was a fair question, and it made me think.

For many years, eating was my way of coping. Like a lot of people, when I felt hurt or confused or abandoned, I found solace in food. Eating was an emotional response to my problems, and it became a habitual response. I didn't know how to communicate and ask for what I wanted. I just accepted what happened to come my way. Food distracted me from feeling empty—it literally filled me up.

Of course, these weren't conscious thoughts at the time. What I realize now is that the decisions I was making about my life then were based on what I thought I deserved. In many ways, it was as if I was viewing the world and responding to it from a child's perspective. While the weight was affecting my adult body and adult life, I think it's possible that my problems with food stemmed from my reactions to situations from childhood—and from the way I perceived them as a child. It was as if I had never outgrown that perspective.

But that didn't change the fact that my fat was real and had become a real problem that I needed to deal with. *The Biggest Loser* provided the gift of a safe environment for me not only to change my body and get healthy, but also to reflect on the emotional responses and decisions that had gotten me to such an unhealthy place.

So I guess the answer to that gentleman's question is: I don't *need* to be protected anymore. I am no longer a child. As I lost the weight, I gained maturity. As an adult, I can see situations and the actions of others for what they really are—and honestly determine whether they have anything to do with me. I'm not a little girl who feels bad about herself. I understand that I'm not responsible for all the unpleasant things that happen in life. It's not about me.

For me, and for a lot of people, weight loss is about so much more than dropping pounds. It is also a journey of personal growth and responsibility. I truly believe that we all have the ability to choose how we *respond* to life. We just have to be willing to take a hard, honest look at ourselves and believe that what we want is within our reach.

BETTE-SUE

I gave my mom a copy of this book when it was still a rough manuscript. I wanted to know what she thought, and I wanted her to be prepared for some of the things I was sharing about our lives. I know that reading it was hard for her. We each needed to take some space and cool down before we could sit down together and talk about it.

Over the years, my mom and I both created situations that we weren't proud of. Our life was never picture perfect, but then again, I don't think that's the reality for most people. The truth is, we are the people we are as a result of all the things that happen to us, good and bad. And for me, my biggest, most influential relationship in life is the one I share with my mother.

Mom was a kid herself when she had Amber and me. I truly believe that Mom did the best she could to raise us, and she would never intentionally hurt her kids. I'm grateful for the many wonderful opportunities she exposed me to, like swimming, a religious foundation that I respect, and her support of our personal growth and reflection. The funny thing is that as an adult, I realize that she and I are more alike than I ever wanted to admit. But do you know what? I can't think of a better person to be like. We are both women who are trying to grow and learn and find ourselves in this world.

The big difference in our relationship now—and it's something that was revisited through the process of writing this book—is that we have learned, and keep learning, to listen to each other. We don't have to accept the blame or guilt or responsibility for one another's pain—we just need to allow each other to express what we feel, and really hear it without becoming defensive or argumentative. Now, when we do clash (and, given our strong personalities, I think some clashing is inevitable!), we bounce back much faster. There are no longer days and weeks that go by when we don't speak to one another. She's a woman, just like me, trying to lead a good life, striving to achieve self-love and self-worth.

Today, my mom is more open than I've ever seen. She's finding pure happiness for herself in her marriage and her affiliation with the Mormon church. I respect what the church fulfills for her and others, and I'm grateful that it brings her such comfort and joy. My mom also *loves* being a grandmother! I think spending time with her grandkids has been healing for her.

We have both grown over the past couple of years. And even though this book temporarily became another hurdle in our relationship, we overcame it. These days there's a sense of calmness to my fiery mom that I've never witnessed before. I think we've both realized that just because we've experienced pain in our lives—sometimes at the hands of one another—that doesn't mean it has to define who we are moving forward. We have the opportunity to choose again every day and make decisions we can be proud of.

As I began this book, so I end it. What I know to be true is that you just have to start putting one foot in front of the other, making an effort to get healthy every day. Over time you'll figure out what motivates you, and you'll find reasons for putting in the hard work required to make changes in your life. It's not always easy to stick with it, but the more you see results, the more clarity you'll start to gain. To think about your life is to create it. You have to take ownership of where you are right now and know where you want to go before you can get there. Keep collecting evidence for your success. You can believe it, and you can be it. Start right now.

Journal Entry

Written While Flying Back to Phoenix after the Finale

My whole life, I have read about and witnessed amazing people accomplishing incredible things, and I look to them for inspiration and confidence. If they can do it, I can do it. Or can I? Am I really a role model? Do I have the strength it takes? Why do I want this? I want to be proud of who I am; I want to honor my parents and my family by honoring myself. I want to show America that you can choose again. I want people to look at me and believe in themselves; I want to own my greatness. I want those lives I come in contact with to be better off having touched mine. I want to believe in good again. I want to prove that it's not a naive mind that believes in greatness but a gutsy one.

I want to empower others through empowering myself. I want to prove that the impossible is possible. That a journey of 1,000 miles really does start with just one step, just one, and that anybody who can imagine that journey does have the strength and courage it takes to pick their foot up and take that first step. I want to know that courage is the light within me that will strengthen and guide me in all of my journeys to come. My body is my Olympic solo, my Tour de France, my Mount Everest, my Super Bowl touchdown, my step on the moon. We all know what dreams are, but do we have the courage and the strength to dream them, to dream impossible dreams, to say, "Yes, I do. Why not, if I am the creator of my destiny and my reality, why not create greatness so that in this moment I choose again?"

I want to make a difference in my community, I want to give, I want to love, I want to have fun, I want to laugh, and I want everybody to do it with me. And I know that in order to really feel happiness, you have to have moments of true sadness . . . I will continue to have those moments, too. But I'll pick myself up every day and brush myself off if need be, knowing that every day is a new day.

The Ali Vincent Stat Sheet

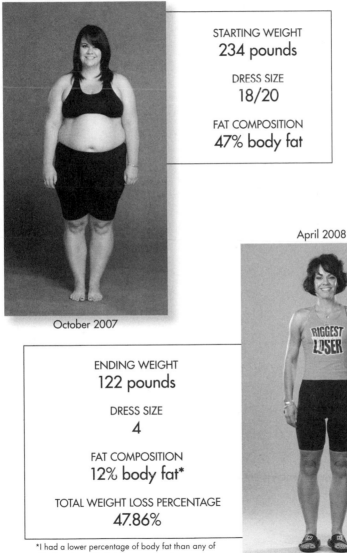

STARTING WEIGHT
234 pounds

DRESS SIZE
18/20

FAT COMPOSITION
47% body fat

October 2007

April 2008

ENDING WEIGHT
122 pounds

DRESS SIZE
4

FAT COMPOSITION
12% body fat*

TOTAL WEIGHT LOSS PERCENTAGE
47.86%

*I had a lower percentage of body fat than any of the American Gladiators, except one!

Notes from Cheryl Forberg, RD, Nutritionist for *The Biggest Loser*

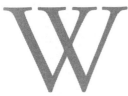hen I applied for *The Biggest Loser,* the show's nutritionist, Cheryl Forberg, RD, took notes about my eating habits. After I won, I asked her if she'd kept her notes on me—I wanted to see them. Whew! They weren't so good. But it only goes to show how much you can change.

Here are her observations from our initial consultation.

Overall

- Salts her food
- Says her diet is "high" in fast food
- Favorite foods: candies and pretzels, lots of snacks
- Very irregular eating patterns
- 8 cups of coffee per day
- 2 liters of diet soft drinks per day
- Little to no water
- 1 serving of vegetables per day: the lettuce and tomato in her fast-food taco
- Eats fruit less than once a day

Typical Workday

- Makes coffee at home
- Goes to Starbucks for a grande nonfat triple shot two-Splenda non-foam latte

Starts Work

- Couple of sodas
- Always chocolates, candy bar miniatures, a few handfuls of pretzels

4:00 p.m.

- Jack in the Box cheeseburger deluxe, tacos
- Two large orders of french fries
- Soda
- Eats all within 10 minutes
- Back to work until 8:00 p.m.
- Drinks coffee or soda

Dinner

- McDonald's two-cheeseburger meal deal with six-piece chicken McNuggets
- Or instead, for dinner with friend, may split a large pizza, jalapeño poppers, and salad
- Lemon drop martini with sugar rim or blood orange margaritas
- And sometimes no dinner, just drinks with friends

Ali's Easy Recipes

I don't like to cook every day, so I've created some fast dishes that work for me. Most of them will make more than one meal (or enough for a meal and a snack). Since I love Mexican food, a lot of my dishes incorporate spicy flavors.

I'm certainly not a chef or culinary expert; I just like making healthy food that tastes delicious. These casual recipes are really just recommendations—they can be modified or adjusted to make something that tastes great to you!

TACOS

I love my tacos! And with this healthy version, I can eat them as often as I want.

> 1 onion, chopped
> 1 clove garlic, chopped
> 2 tablespoons salsa
> Ground cumin, to taste
> 1 pound extra-lean ground turkey
> 3 corn tortillas

In a nonstick skillet, cook the onion, garlic, salsa, and cumin. Add the ground turkey and cook until browned.

Warm the tortillas in the oven until they're crisp. Spoon 4 ounces of the mixture into each tortilla. Top with tomatoes, lettuce or cabbage, and more salsa.

Variations:

Sometimes I substitute diced boneless, skinless chicken breasts for the turkey. I also make a variation that includes zucchini when I use chicken breast.

Instead of salsa, sometimes I substitute a spicy Mexican tomato sauce called El Taco. It comes in a yellow can.

BLACK BEANS AND NOT-RICE

These simple and inexpensive ingredients provide a lot of fiber and protein. I buy canned organic black beans and rinse them.

2 cups quinoa
1 can black beans, rinsed
Salsa
Chopped fresh cilantro

Cook the quinoa according to the package directions and stir in the beans. Top with salsa and cilantro. This recipe makes two servings.

ORZO PASTA WITH CHICKEN

This easy dish satisfies my pasta cravings and packs a protein punch.

Whole wheat orzo or other whole wheat pasta
Boneless, skinless chicken tenders, cut into bite-size pieces
Lemon juice
Chopped fresh cilantro

Cook the pasta according to the package directions—I usually make a large batch, a few cups. Cook the chicken tenders in a nonstick skillet coated with cooking spray. (I use Pam.) Season with salt-free seasonings, like those from Mrs. Dash.

For one serving, I measure out 3 to 4 ounces of cooked chicken and ½ cup of pasta. Sprinkle with a little lemon juice and cilantro. Yum!

PITA SANDWICH

Nothing beats a good veggie-loaded sandwich for lunch!

½ whole wheat pita
3 ounces cooked boneless, skinless chicken breast
¼ cup alfalfa sprouts
¼ cup chopped cucumber
½ cup chopped tomato
¼ avocado

Stuff the half pita with the chicken, sprouts, cucumber, tomato, and avocado and season as desired—I add lots of fresh black pepper.

BREAKFAST SANDWICH

I used to buy greasy breakfast sandwiches back in my drive-thru days. This version is vastly improved and just as tasty!

1 egg
1 slice turkey bacon
1 whole wheat English muffin, toasted
1 slice low-fat cheese

In a nonstick skillet coated with cooking spray, fry the egg. Add the turkey bacon to the same pan and cook until browned.

Transfer the egg and bacon to the bottom half of the toasted muffin and top with the cheese, then add the muffin top. The heat from all the surrounding ingredients will melt the cheese and form a nice, gooey breakfast sandwich.

SCRAMBLED EGGS

I love this quick, easy, and flavorful breakfast. It's virtually fat free and very low in calories.

> **4 egg whites**
> **Salsa**
> **1 wedge Laughing Cow light cheese**

In a nonstick skillet coated with cooking spray, cook the egg whites. When they're almost done, add a few spoonfuls of salsa and the wedge of cheese. Cook, stirring, over medium heat until the eggs are cooked, the salsa is warmed, and the cheese begins to melt. Eat immediately.

FRUIT AND OATMEAL

This sweet breakfast is a great way to get calcium and vitamin C, and it will keep you full all morning long!

> **Instant oatmeal**
> **Fat-free milk**
> **5 or 6 strawberries, chopped**
> **¼ cup blueberries**
> **¼ banana, chopped**
> **Cinnamon**

Cook the oatmeal according to the package directions, using milk instead of water. Stir in the fruit and sprinkle with a little bit of cinnamon.